The Ultimate Guide
to Sex and Disability

ABOUT THE AUTHORS

MIRIAM KAUFMAN, M.D., is a pediatrician and adolescent health specialist at the Hospital for Sick Children in Toronto and an Associate Professor at the University of Toronto. She is the author of *Easy for You to Say: Q&A's for Teens Living with Chronic Illness or Disability* and *Overcoming Teen Depression: A Guide for Parents,* co-author of *Your Overweight Child: Promoting Fitness and Self-Esteem,* and is the editor of *Mothering Teens: Understanding the Adolescent Years.* She is a regular speaker at conferences and has been interviewed by *The New York Times, Time Magazine* and many other newspapers and magazines. She has appeared on television and radio, including The Oprah Winfrey Show and the CBC. She graduated from Duke University School of Nursing and Queen's University Faculty of Medicine.

CORY SILVERBERG, M.Ed., is a founding member Come As You Are, a co-operatively run, education based sex store in Toronto. He has conducted workshops across North America on sex toys, sexual communication, and sexuality and disability. He is a media consultant and a regular contributor in the national media on the subject of sexuality. He received his Masters of Education specializing in counseling psychology from the University of Toronto.

FRAN ODETTE, MSW, is a project coordinator with the Women with Disabilities and Violence Initiative at Education Wife Assault in Toronto. She is the former Project Coordinator of SexAbility: A Program of Planned Parenthood of Toronto in partnership with the Anne Johnston Health Station. She has presented on the topics of women's health, body image, sexual health, and disability across Canada and the U.S. She received her Masters in Social Work from Carlton University.

The Ultimate Guide to Sex and Disability

FOR ALL OF US WHO LIVE WITH DISABILITIES,
CHRONIC PAIN, AND ILLNESS

by Miriam Kaufman, M.D.,
Cory Silverberg, and Fran Odette

Illustrated by Fiona Smyth

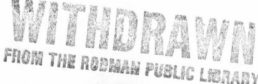

CLEIS
PRESS

Published in the United States by Cleis Press Inc.,
P.O. Box 14684, San Francisco, California 94114.

Printed in the United States.
Cover design: Scott Idleman
Book design: Karen Quigg
Cleis Press logo art: Juana Alicia
First Edition.
10 9 8 7 6 5 4 3 2 1

Bob Flanagan quote taken from *Bob Flanagan: Supermasochist,* edited by A. Juno & V. Vale
(Re/Search Publications, 1993).

Library of Congress Cataloging-in-Publication Data

Kaufman, Miriam.
  The ultimate guide to sex and disability: for all of us who live with disabilities, chronic pain,
and illness / by Miriam Kaufman, Fran Odette, and Cory Silverberg.— 1st ed.
      p. cm.
  ISBN 1-57344-176-7 (alk. paper)
  1. Chronically ill—Sexual behavior. 2. Handicapped—Sexual behavior.
  3. People with disabilities—Sexual behavior. 4. Sex instruction for people with disabilities.
  I. Odette, Fran. II. Silverberg, Cory. III. Title.
    RC108.K38 2003
    613.9'5'087—dc22

                                                            2003010510

To the memory of

Barbara Waxman Fiducia

Acknowledgments

First and foremost we want to thank all the people who participated in our survey. Their words guided the content of this book and gave it a spirit far beyond what we could have done ourselves. Thanks also go to our professional readers Sharon Vilcini, Ann Barrett, and Barry Siskind who waded through a much longer, more chaotic version of this book and made it leaner and more thoughtful.

The work of many colleagues (some of whom we have never met) has inspired us as we put this book together. Thanks in this regard to Michael Barrett, Linda Crabtree, Dominic Davies, Kath Duncan, Anne Finger, Dave Hingsburger, Paul Longmore, Susan Ludwig, Nancy Mairs, Linda Mona, Corbett O'Toole, Tuppy Owens, Kenneth Ray Stubbs, Mitch Tepper, and Rebecca Widom.

Special thanks to our friends and colleagues who helped out directly in countless ways: Anne Amitay, Rosemary Antze, Chloe Atkins, Roberta Benson, Jennifer Bator, Joani Blank, Viviana Cornejo, Athena Douris, Sarah Forbes-Roberts, Pat Israel, Jasmine Lefresne, Aruna Mitra, Robert Morgan, Caroline O'Reilly, Rebecca Pitcherack, Carol Queen, Anne Semans, Mary Sutherland, Cathy Winks, Hilde Zitzelsberger, the producers of "Sex TV," and the worker-owners of Come As You Are and Good Vibrations.

Finally, we have to thank Felice Newman and Frédérique Delacoste from Cleis Press. They approached us to produce this book and showed infinite patience with three authors who have too many day jobs. We thank them for their enthusiasm, support, and their ongoing commitment to publish books that need to be published.

Contents

ix   **Introduction**

1   *CHAPTER 1:* **Myths About Disability and Sex**

13   *CHAPTER 2:* **Desire and Self-Esteem**

27   *CHAPTER 3:* **Sexual Anatomy and Sexual Response**

69   *CHAPTER 4:* **Communication**

110   *CHAPTER 5:* **Sex with Ourselves**

124   *CHAPTER 6:* **Sex with Others**

150   *CHAPTER 7:* **Oral Sex**

168   *CHAPTER 8:* **Penetration and Positioning**

185   *CHAPTER 9:* **Sex Toys, Books, and Videos**

223   *CHAPTER 10:* **Yoga and Tantric Sex**

234   *CHAPTER 11:* **S/M**

256   *CHAPTER 12:* **Sexual Health**

274   *CHAPTER 13:* **Sexual Violence and Sexuality**

290   *CHAPTER 14:* **Resources**

329   *CHAPTER 15:* **Glossary of Gender and Sex Terms**

335   **Index**

Illustrations

1. Respiratory System, page 35
2. Female Anatomy, External, page 40
3. Female Anatomy, Internal, page 43
4. Male Anatomy, External, page 44
5. Male Anatomy, Internal, page 46
6. Products to Use for Kegel Exercises, page 60
7. Position: Partner on Top, page 179
8. Position: Using Wheelchair, page 181
9. Position: Side-by-Side, page 182
10. Position: Using Furniture, page 183
11. Vibrators, page 193
12. Dildos, page 196
13. Anal Toys, page 199

Abbreviations Used in This Book

AAC   Augmentative and Alternative Communication

AD   Autonomic Dysreflexia

ALS   Amyotrophic Lateral Sclerosis

CF   Cystic Fibrosis

CP   Cerebral Palsy

GLBT   Gay, Lesbian, Bisexual, Transgendered/Transsexual

MD   Muscular Dystrophy

MS   Multiple Sclerosis

PCA   Personal Care Attendant

PTSD   Post-Traumatic Stress Disorder

SCI   Spinal Cord Injury

STI/STD   Sexually Transmitted Infection/ Sexually Transmitted Disease

TAB   Temporarily Abled-Bodied

Introduction

To realize our sexual freedom, our goal must be to infuse the dominant sexual culture with the richness of our own experience. We must celebrate our differences from those without disabilities. We must see that our differences in appearance and function which are the sources of our degradation also contain the seeds of our sexual liberation.
—BARBARA FAYE WAXMAN, "It's Time to Politicize Our Sexual Oppression," The Disability Rag, March/April 1991

The ULTIMATE *Guide to Sex and Disability*? Just who do we think we are, anyway?

Well, we don't think we, or anyone else, could actually write the ultimate guide, if by that we mean a book that says everything that could be said and contains information about every conceivable disability and chronic illness. Instead, we think that each person needs to "write" their own *Ultimate Guide to My Sexuality*, and then update it regularly.

This book helps you do precisely that. It pulls together the available information on sex and disability that isn't aimed at a particular disability. While many of the issues in this book are unique to disability, the larger experience of trying to define one's own sexual life is not.

Much of the information in this book comes from our professional work, our interactions with colleagues and clients, and things that have been written in the past. A lot of it comes from our personal experiences with friends and lovers. But what made up the foundation of this book were the responses we got to a survey about sex that we distributed to people living with disabilities. While the other information we've collected is important and we hope it will be helpful, by far the most interesting and informative part of writing this book has been reading and incorporating the survey responses. Our highly unscientific survey was distributed via the Internet and also by telephone. We asked people twelve very open-ended questions about a variety of aspects of sexuality. The responses were amazing and wide-ranging, and those people who didn't like our questions told us so and made up their own instead.

The survey participants whose words enrich so much of this book have a great deal to teach people living with, and without, disabilities and chronic illnesses. Our respondents live with a wide range of mobility, sensory, environmental, developmental, cognitive, and psychiatric disabilities.

We hope this book will generate ideas for you, start conversations among the important people in your life, let you share in the wisdom of those who took our survey, and point you to the rich lode of practical information we found.

In writing this book we often struggled with language. There are three of us: One of us lives with a disability, one has a chronic condition, and the third is currently nondisabled. We decided to use the inclusive "we" when referring to people with disabilities. We see ourselves as people who struggle with our own issues of difference and who are working to identify with the challenges that our readers face every day. We wrote this book for anyone who is interested in sex. You don't have to have a sexual partner, or even be thinking about getting one. We haven't aimed it at those who are a particular gender, or have a particular sexual orientation, or live with a particular disability. Although most of the people who read our book will identify themselves as living with a disability, or chronic pain or illness, we expect that nondisabled partners, parents, health care providers, other care providers, and teachers will be interested as well.

Because we know this book isn't the final word on sex and disability, we have compiled one of the most extensive collections ever of user-friendly resources on sexuality and disability. We list books, organizational contacts, and plenty of websites. While we don't discuss reproduction or pregnancy, you'll find resources in chapter 14 that can help you access information on these topics.

We have included exercises you can try at the end of many of the chapters. The exercises might allow some people to take a few moments to consider what they've read in the chapter and how it reflects their own life. In addition to working on them on your own, they may help you start talking about sexuality and disability with a friend, counselor, or someone else whom you trust in your life.

A little about us.... Cory is a founding member of Come As You Are, a worker-owned, cooperative sex toy store and website in Toronto, Canada (www.comeasyouare.com). The retail store is a fully accessible, disability-positive space. Cory has also worked as a sex educator in various disability and rehabilitation communities for the past nine years. As someone who is currently nondisabled, most of his work has been with other nondisabled professionals, teaching them to be more comfortable talking about sexuality. His work has also focused on adapting sex toys to meet various needs. Cory has a master's degree in psychology and has conducted academic research on sexuality and disability.

Fran is a queer gal living with a mobility disability. She has been working in the areas of sexuality and disability for a number of years, mostly centered on training and educating of service providers about issues that impact persons living with disabilities, and sexuality and sexual health. Fran has cofacilitated workshops for women living with disabilities on aspects of body image, sexuality, and disability. She is a contributor to "dis-n-tangle," a 'zine for lesbian/gay/bisexual/transgendered/transsexual folks living with disabilities and our allies. Previously, Fran was the coordinator of SexAbility, a program of Planned Parenthood in Toronto (in partnership with the Anne Johnston Health Station). This program offers sexual health information and workshops to youth living with disabilities.

Miriam is a pediatrician and specialist in Adolescent Medicine at The Hospital for Sick Children in Toronto, as well as an associate professor at the University of Toronto. Miriam has a chronic endocrine condition but is not disabled by it. She got interested in sex education while a nursing student at Duke University, and has been involved in the field ever since. A major part of Miriam's work is in public education. For the past three years she wrote a weekly teen advice column in a daily newspaper and has written two books, edited one, and coauthored another. Her favorite (alas, out of print) is *Easy for You to Say: Q & A's for Teens Living with Chronic Illness or Disability.* She is a lesbian who lives with her partner of more than twenty-five years and their two teenaged children.

Fran and Cory met almost eight years ago through sex education work they were doing in the community. Miriam then met the two of them while presenting a workshop for young people with spina bifida. Writing this book has given the three of us a wonderful opportunity to become friends.

Sexual independence is an extremely potent form of empowerment. It is our belief (and our personal experience) that by exploring our sexuality, by deciding that we are worthy of feeling pleasure and of realizing our possibilities as sexual beings, we can change other parts of our lives as well. We hope that this book will lead to positive changes in the lives of you, our readers, and in turn will create a ripple effect, building a movement of sexual liberation for those of us living with disabilities and chronic conditions; for our allies, lovers, and partners; and, most importantly, for ourselves.

Miriam Kaufman, M.D.
Cory Silverberg
Fran Odette
Toronto, September 2003

1

Myths About Disability and Sexuality

Why begin a sex guide with what isn't true about sex and sexuality? We do so because wrong ideas about sex and disability affect us all. Many of these ideas have been communicated in such subtle ways that we aren't even aware that we believe them. When we *do* believe them, we limit our possibilities as sexual beings and damage our self-esteem. And when other people believe them, their perspectives on us as people with disabilities are based on these mistruths, and in turn they see us inaccurately as asexual or fragile and are not interested in us as sexual partners.

We want to discuss these myths in an effort to deactivate them—to wipe the slate clean before presenting information over the course of the book that dispels these myths.

Myth #1: People living with disabilities and chronic illnesses are not sexual.

Once or twice a year, a journalist "discovers" the idea of sexuality and disability and decides it will make a great human interest story. Other than this, we rarely find media depictions of people living with disabilities or chronic illnesses as having sex lives. And if we do, it is usually presented as a rare and incredible thing.

We think this happens for two reasons. First is the belief of many nondisabled people that they themselves will never become disabled. By distancing themselves from all things related to disability, they manage to stay in denial. Second is the fact that many nondisabled people view people living with disabilities as essentially different from them. They think we are helpless (because we may need help) and therefore are like children, who are not acknowledged to be sexual. You may have sixty years' life experience, with the body, brain, temperament, and libido of an adult, but if you can't feed yourself, or need help wiping your ass, or getting in and out of the car, you are considered a child. Thus they deny our sexualities.

In North American culture, self-sufficiency is highly prized, defined as the ability to do everything for yourself—and still have energy left over to help those poor unfortunates who are not as self-sufficient as you! It is not defined as the ability to work creatively and cooperatively with others.

Myth #2: People living with disabilities and chronic illnesses are not desirable.

We've all been fed the message that sex is for the young and beautiful. If you don't resemble a twenty-three-year-old supermodel, no one will want you. Likewise, if you cannot produce multiple G-spot orgasms on cue or perform like a stud, you're not worth going to bed with.

This standard exists for us all, and harms us all. Even worse is the notion that if you require some help with assistive devices, or a little extra patience, communication, and emotional support before you can enjoy giving and receiving sexual pleasure, you're a burden. Who would want you?

Myth #3: Sex must be spontaneous.

We're taught that sex is supposed to be spontaneous, something that just comes naturally (like "true love"). This belief is damaging to everyone, but is a real problem for people living with disabilities, because any amount of planning makes sex *not* spontaneous. Believing in this myth pretty much ensures a lousy sex life.

While sex has many meanings, at its heart sex is a process of communication. Whether we are flirting from across a crowded room, giving someone head for the first time, or making love while listening to a piece of music that totally turns us on, being sexual is being in contact with ourselves and our surroundings. The idea that this process can happen without thinking, talking, or planning is ridiculous.

Maybe we are willing to buy into the myth of sexual spontaneity because talking about our desires is difficult. It's risky, and makes us feel exposed and vulnerable, and often vulnerability is equated with weakness.

Myth #4: People who live with disabilities and chronic illnesses can't have "real" sex.

Watch any one of the thousands of mainstream porn films (or even regular films with sex scenes) released each year and you'll get some idea of how sex is "supposed" to work. "Real" sex progresses from light activities like kissing to the "real" thing, penis-in-vagina intercourse, to simultaneous orgasm in ten minutes or less. You should also be able to have sex in a variety of different positions all in the same night. Everything we do sexually is supposed to progress toward that goal, and none of it is as important as the result itself. Thus "foreplay" is nothing more than a prelude to the main event. Oral sex is hot, but it's still not as good as the "real" thing.

According to this way of thinking, masturbation doesn't count as sex. Only people who can't get laid masturbate. Of course, studies (not to mention our own experience!) tell us this is not true. People of all genders and sexual orientations, whether single, partnered, or multipartnered, masturbate! Some of us even masturbate with our partners.

Most of us are raised with at least a few negative messages about pleasing ourselves sexually, one of which is that orgasms experienced alone aren't as fulfilling as those had with a partner. Unfortunately, the taboo against self-pleasure is deeply ingrained in us. And this taboo flares to a fevered pitch if someone needs help to get off on their own.

So only intercourse leading to orgasm is considered "real sex," and within that idea lies a belief that no one living with a disability is capable of having intercourse. The truth is that the majority of us *can* have intercourse, and those of us who can't, or choose not to, can still have real sex.

Myth #5: People living with disabilities and chronic illnesses are pathetic choices for partners.

This reveals a deep bias: If you live with a disability or serious illness, you must be a pitiable creature, and if I feel so poorly about you, you must feel worse about yourself. And why would I want to choose a lover with such a lousy self-image?

The even more dangerous underlying idea is that if you live with a disability, whatever you happen to feel about yourself or think about the world on a particular day must be related to your disability. If you're a real complainer who likes to kvetch and make everyone's life miserable, it surely is because you have a disability. On the other hand, if you are always cheerful, looking on the positive side of things, that too must be indicative of what a trouper you are, to be happy in spite of living such a terrible existence. Of course, we all have good days and bad days. But when you live with a visible disability or chronic illness, whatever you are on a given day is believed to be *a result of* your condition.

Related to this is the deeply disturbing idea that living with a disability is a life not worth living. We're taught to feel sorry for anyone who cannot achieve "good" health (basically, the absence of any condition that makes you different from anyone else). If we believe that people who live with disabilities are helpless, powerless, unnatural burdens, then few options are open to us, and none of them involve being in a satisfying sexual relationship.

> When I was in my twenties, I got engaged to a nondisabled guy. My family freaked because they couldn't understand what this guy saw in me and thought that whatever he saw in me wouldn't last. My family felt that being with me would be a novelty and eventually the novelty would wear off and he would lose interest in me because how can someone like me be a good "wife" to him... especially sexually?

Myth #6: People living with disabilities and chronic illnesses have more important things than sex to worry about.

Who says sex isn't important? Well, just about everyone in a position to teach us about sex manages to subtly convey the message that sex is a frivolous pastime, certainly not something responsible citizens need, unless we're talking about the serious business of procreation.

The point is made again and again that if you live with a disability or chronic illness you've got more important things to deal with. Sex is a luxury you simply can't afford. This is also tied into the idea that people living with disabilities are childlike and need to be told how to prioritize their lives. This attitude is held by many nondisabled people, and even certain disability-rights activists claim that talking about our individual issues is bad because it "fragments the cause."

Myth #7: People living with disabilities and chronic illnesses are not sexually adventurous.

and

Myth #8: People living with disabilities and chronic illnesses who have sex are perverts.

These myths are two sides of the same coin. On the one side, if you look as if you live with a disability, it is assumed that you are passive. This assumption is generalized to all areas in our lives. It is taken for granted that people living with disabilities are sexually passive and noninitiators. People can't imagine that someone who uses a wheelchair might want to be tied up and spanked, or that a man with no legs gets off dressing up as a ballerina. A second layer of meaning related to this myth is the idea that all anyone wants is to be just like everyone else. So to those of us who are seen as different in some major way, it is particularly important that we pass as "normal." We all know that "normal" people don't like to dress up or get spanked, right?

The "pervert" myth, the flip side of the same coin, paints a picture of the dirty old man with the cane eyeing all the young, nubile whatevers in the park. Ageism and disability often go hand in hand in the way they marginalize people. Underlying both these myths is the notion that people living with disabilities and chronic illnesses are "other" and that for them to have any interest in sex is perverted.

Myth #9: We all get what we deserve, and we can always do more to help ourselves.

Whether we believe in karma or a simple do-unto-others philosophy for daily living, most of us are taught to believe that good things will happen to good people and bad things to bad people. Thus it follows that if you have HIV, use a wheelchair to get around, or have trouble breathing, then you must have done something to deserve it. If we believe bad things happen to bad people, we then don't have to imagine the possibility of a similar reality for ourselves.

So if we are experiencing too much pain to enjoy sex, there must be a reason. This irritating message often comes in the form of well-meaning suggestions from friends and family about doctors, chiropractors, naturopaths, herbalists, massage therapists, talk therapists, and others. Maybe we should try this, or that, and then we'll be better, or perhaps even okay. This is no different from the habit most of us have of blaming the victim, by wondering or overtly asking "Are you really doing enough to change your situation?"

The reality is that no matter how much we love ourselves, no matter how skilled we become at negotiating the particulars of our self-care, some of us experience physical pain that won't go away. That pain becomes a fact of our lives. With life often comes pain—as unacceptable as this idea is to many people.

Myth #10: People living in institutions shouldn't have sex.

One of the greatest barriers many people living with disabilities face when trying to develop a positive sexuality is a lack of privacy. Nowhere is this more evident than in institutions like rehab hospitals, hospices, group homes, and nursing homes. Most such institutions systematically deny residents the right to be sexual, whether alone or with others. No locks on doors; no privacy; the right of staff to treat people as objects to be carted around, talked about in the third person even in their presence, and controlled—these are just a few of the ways that institutions make it clear that sexuality is not acceptable. The underlying belief is that people's behaviors must be monitored because they are incapable of monitoring themselves.

> Living in an institution means that I have no privacy. I have a crush on the guy who lives here and some of the staff found out. Well now they are always making comments about "how cute it is" when we are together. When he and I have a chance to be alone

in my room listening to music, we might be cuddling or holding hands while we're in our wheelchairs. I don't know how many times the staff come and knock on the door, telling us that "doors must be open at all times" unless the staff are in here with us. I hate it and I feel that I don't have anyone here that understands how alone I feel.

This leads us to another myth.

Myth #11: Sex is private.

If we were taught anything about sex at all when we were younger, many of us learned that sex was something private, inappropriate to talk about or do in front of others. Privacy becomes a requirement for sexuality.

For someone living in an institution, or using attendant services, or needing the assistance of someone else to facilitate communication, privacy is a completely different reality. The definition of privacy changes when you have no lock on your door, or when you request private time at a specific hour knowing that it will probably be written down in a log-book. This myth is one of those "no-win situations," because we're told that real sex is a private matter and, guess what, you can't have that kind of privacy.

Myth #12: People living with disabilities and chronic illnesses don't get sexually assaulted.

If you aren't seen as sexually desirable in our culture, you won't get sexually assaulted, right? Wrong. People who live with physical disabilities are far more likely to be victims of sexual assault than those who don't live with physical disabilities. Some statistics suggest that people living with disabilities are two to ten times more likely to be assaulted than those who do not have disabilities. This abuse ranges from pervasive power abuses by medical and rehabilitation staff to rape and other forms of sexual assault, forced confinement, physical abuse, and more. Supports for disclosure of the abuse, legal action, and counseling are scarce for people living with disabilities. This is especially true in institutions that maintain a culture of secrecy and keeping things private, which in turn allows more opportunities for other forms of abuse.

This myth sets up one of the most horrific, self-perpetuating cycles: If you are not at risk, why bother creating programs for prevention and support? This attitude places you at greater risk, and the cycle continues.

Myth #13: People living with disabilities and chronic illnesses don't need sex education.

The false beliefs we are outlining in this chapter tend to build on each other. So, if we aren't considered sexual, then there is no reason for us to get sex education. Sexual ignorance is an enormous obstacle for all of us when trying to figure ourselves out sexually. Our situation is made worse when we are systematically denied access to the little bit of sex education most people get.

Another layer of this idea is the belief that if you tell someone about sex they will immediately become fucking machines. And few things scare the nondisabled public more than the idea of people living with disabilities reproducing. This is especially true for people who live with intellectual and developmental disabilities. For those of us living with other types of disabilities, we also face huge obstacles to having children. Part of what motivates people to deny sex education programs to people living with disabilities is the perception that such programs will open up a can of worms, which the nondisabled professionals will "have to deal with" because those of us living with disabilities will be incapable of handling it responsibly and it will become someone else's problem.

With very few exceptions, sex education programs designed for people living with disabilities take a cookie-cutter approach to sexual response: If you have an SCI at such and such a level, then *this* model is what you can expect for your sexuality. If you're seventy years old and just had a stroke, then your sexuality will look like *this*.

In this book we take a fundamentally different approach. We want to help you become the expert about your own sexuality.

Myth #14: People living with disabilities and chronic illnesses are unnatural.

My level of dependency presents me as a "passenger" in other people's eyes.

This is the same us-versus-them dichotomy that society maintains in regard to sex, race, religion, and all the other ways that people differ from one another. Lots of different ideas have been floated about why it's so important to maintain this difference when it comes to disability and illness. Some say people are ashamed of the way nondisabled culture has treated people living with disabilities. This shame makes it hard for the nondisabled to start seeing "us" as really being part of "them" because that would mean acknowledging all the horrible things "they" have done to "us" (confusing, isn't it?). Others say the reason is nondisabled people's fear of pain, suffering, and death—all the things that are equated with disability and illness. Whatever the reason, it is clear that many nondisabled people have a lot invested in maintaining this distinction.

Aside from all the obvious ways in which this myth is used to justify segregating people living with disabilities from society, it's interesting to notice how this myth also defines disability as that which we can easily recognize. Many disabilities and chronic illnesses are "invisible." If you live with endometriosis, or you've just been diagnosed with MS, or you have chronic fatigue, or are hard of hearing, you don't really fit into either category. You may *feel* disabled, but nondisabled people will treat you like one of their own because you look "fine." So where do you fit in?

I have chronic fatigue and for most people who first meet me, they have no idea. This is a real issue when going out on dates for the first time and trying to figure out "when do I tell them about this?," especially if they want to plan something that will require a lot of energy such as dancing or some other type of physical activity.

Initially, most people are okay with it in the beginning, but when it starts to interfere with their "fun" then it becomes an issue. It's hard for them to understand the times when I'm feeling good and we are able to do things together, to then to see me suddenly crash and need to hibernate for a few days and not do anything. Sometimes they take it personally or get frustrated. Some relationships have ended because I haven't been in the space to negotiate their discomfort.

Some people feel that *not* fitting in with the dominant norm and experiencing life with some sort of "difference" is in fact a great benefit, because it both releases them from the expectations of others and allows them to look at themselves in new ways.

In our culture we are bombarded with messages about who we are supposed to be, how we are supposed to act, and what our lives are supposed to mean. Therefore it's hard to separate the expectations that have been placed on us from our own feelings and needs. This is especially true about sexuality. In the following chapters, we will offer specific ways to liberate our sex lives from the limitations of these damaging myths and unrealistic expectations.

It took work as a teenager to reconcile my version of who I am with the world's version of who I am. Now, I live with my version, though occasionally that collides with the world's perceptions. For example, if someone hands me money on the street, I could interpret the gesture as their belief that I am impoverished and unable to earn a living; however, my version of it is that they are paying me for brightening up their day with my charm. Okay—I am being tongue-in-cheek here, but my point is that I prefer to change what I can that I don't like, but let the rest roll off my back. I can dwell on those situations that could whittle at my self-esteem or I could say, "Forgive them, they know not what they do." I'm not passive, though—if I think that a person is trainable, I will attempt to educate them. Meanwhile, I am the person in control of how I feel about myself, not others. I chose to keep that power.

Exercises

1. Can you think of a recent situation where you were the brunt of someone's negative beliefs about sex and disability or illness? Was it something said by a friend, family member, or lover? A character in a movie or television show? A look or gesture from a stranger? How did you respond?

2. What about your own biases regarding sex and disability or illness? Do you think disabled people "should" be sexual? What kinds of sexual activities do you think are "normal"? What things do you think are "wrong"? How have your beliefs influenced your interactions with others?

Desire and Self-Esteem

I spent my teen years desperately wanting something, but I didn't know what it was. I didn't think it could be sex, because when I heard other guys talking about girls, it was all about how they looked, and since I can't see girls I figured I couldn't be attracted to them. They never talked about how girls smell, the way a breast feels cupped in your hand, how you feel when they whisper things in your ears, the thrill of kissing.... As you can see, I've got it figured out now, but then it was just a nameless desire.

Before sex, before the thoughts and ideas about sex, comes desire. Desire is a state of longing. More than ordinary wanting, we feel an urgency—we *must* have what we desire. Desire, whether or not it is sexual, is a physical sensation that can be felt as a tugging of the heart as easily as a throbbing in the groin. It can arise from many different stimuli, physical, emotional, and mental. A smell can trigger desire, but so can a sexual fantasy, or an attractive person passing by our window.

Unfortunately, many of us go from desire immediately to all the reasons why what we want is wrong, dirty, or immoral. We may think that it would be acceptable for someone else, but for us it either can't or shouldn't happen. In doing this we immediately shut down our desire.

But a magical moment occurs before we get to the negative thoughts that shut us down: a moment of desire, something we all experience regardless of physical, mental, or emotional disability. Linger in that moment, relish it and the many possibilities it presents.

How Important Are Sex and Desire?

Sexuality fluctuates in its importance in our lives. At times it is not a focus at all—those times when we are wrapped up in other aspects of our lives. At other times, sex is all we think about. Different people have different levels of desire, and we all have different intimacy needs as well.

Sexual desire becomes a problem when we deny we are feeling it. It's when we close ourselves off to the possibility of sexual desire, or when we ignore that desire can be played out in all sorts of ways, that we get ourselves tied up in knots and fail to get what we really want.

Sex has always been and continues to be an important part of my life. My husband and I can be emotionally and physically close in many ways—talking, cuddling, etc.—but there's just no substitute for the intimacy and satisfaction that comes from great sex with the partner you love. Sex isn't the most important thing in life, but it's right up there. I've had bilateral total knee replacements, two different femur fractures (one required me to wear a cast; the other required surgery), and other injuries such as tendonitis. Through it all, my husband and I managed to have sex within days after my surgeries and even with my long-leg cast on! It was challenging but fun and well worth the effort. At times, I have a lot of pain with my arthritis but when I'm having sex, I forget all about it. And the release of endorphins is wonderful!

Self-Image and Self-Esteem

Thousands of books, self-help courses, infomercials, and talk shows have been devoted to self-image and self-esteem. But what do these terms really mean? Self-image is simply your view of yourself. It includes what you think you look like and what kind of a person you think you are. Discrepancies always exist, of course, between how we view ourselves and how others view us. Many of us have a very stable self-image that doesn't change even when our weight, hair color, or skills change. This can be protective, but it can also make change difficult. If you have learned to view yourself as a nonsexual person, it can be hard to start thinking of yourself as sexual or sexy. It may be painful to even consider contemplating yourself in that light.

How I see myself definitely affects my sexuality and vice versa. There are times when I feel very sexy and know that people are interested in me, and those times are great. But I have also gone through long periods with no one asking me out, and I felt completely like this ugly, undesirable person. Over the years I've found some tricks, like getting myself new clothes—in my case they are new used clothes, but new to me! I change my hair A LOT, and try to spend more time with friends, but it can be hard to get out of the rut of feeling like no one is ever going to want to fuck you again. At these times hearing nice things from my friends doesn't really help.

Self-esteem is more complicated, as it involves an implied judgment. It also involves how we feel about our self-image. Some people say that how we feel about ourselves—our self-esteem—can be expressed as the difference between the way that we want people to see us and the way that we think we are.

> *I hate being disabled. Being disabled has stunted my growth, deformed my spine, made me poor. All this affects my self-esteem. Few people are attracted to impoverished, deformed cripples.*

> *There is no doubt that my disability affects my self-esteem, but this is not due to my disability, but because of society's attitude toward those of us who are disabled. We are made to feel like second-class citizens just because we are unable to partake in certain activities or we may look a little different. Just because I live with a disability does not give people the right to stare, point, or laugh at me. Disabled people do have feelings too, and often a lot of people tend to forget this. We are seen as objects that can provide a moment's ridicule for those with very small minds.*

It is very difficult not to internalize negative messages, not to consider ourselves lacking in comparison to the dominant norm. We can do several things to deal with these messages. We can give ourselves more positive messages, and take in compliments when they're given. We can listen to what people who feel good about themselves have to say and use that as a cue to actively speak about ourselves in positive ways. We can try to think about ourselves as attractive, desirable, worthy, and good.

> *Before I became disabled, I was very much into looking good and keeping physically fit. Sex was usually rigorous and spontaneous. But after my injury that changed. I really wasn't sure who I was. I believed that who I was was wrapped up in what my body could do and looked like. It took a long time and a lot of effort to think differently about myself. I still have to catch myself from thinking that I'm not a "real man" because I can't keep up with the boys or have sex like I was used to. Meeting other quads and talking to them about how they were coping let me reevaluate things in my life. I have found that it's easier to just try to be as comfortable as I can with who I am.*

Pain and Self-Esteem

My disability is degenerative, but I'm a woman who really likes to do things for herself. Because of that, when my disability is stable (or even improving, like when I get a better drug) my self-esteem is very high. I set limits that push myself, but won't kill me, do as much as I can, and feel very good about myself. I really feel that I put more energy into caring for myself and my community than a lot of people do, so I don't feel shame in asking for help when I feel that I need it or when it would be very good for me. During my downturns, though, I feel horrendous emotional crashes. I don't know where to set my limits, and I'm afraid of the pain. So I hold back, careful not to push my body into a pain crisis, but I worry constantly the whole time that I'm not doing all I could do.

During my worst downturn, for about six years, the pain was so constant and severe that I could sleep only every third night. Even narcotics helped only a little. Though I had hurt constantly for a long time, during this downturn I lost my ability to focus attention on anything other than the deep pain I could only describe as like a knitting needle being pushed into the ends of my bones, sometimes slowly, sometimes quickly, thrusting through the length of them. I'm still not sure how I managed to hold my constant scream inside my chest. At the time, like in other downturns, my self-esteem plummeted. But now, I gain an immense well of self-esteem from the knowledge that I survived when pain was my whole world and no one, not even any doctor, could promise me that it would ever be different.

Identity and Self-Esteem

A sense of identity includes both knowing who we are independent of the world outside and who we are as part of a larger group or society. Having a strong sense of identity is about being comfortable inside our own skin, belonging to our community. It's one way of knowing for sure that there are other people out there like us, offering confirmation and validation that the way we are is real.

> In general, I'm happy with myself. In fact, much of what I like about myself—graduating college, running for office, being elected, being able to get along with a diverse group of people—is directly related to my being disabled. I always thought that if I hadn't been disabled I would've been a jock. I attribute much of my intellectual accomplishments to being disabled and I'm very proud of those accomplishments.

But if you're not so happy with your self, or your community, taking on a new identity is not always easy or smooth. People often assume that simply by meeting the external requirements of a group you must be a member of that group. For instance, that if you look as if you have a disability, you must identify (think, speak, and act) as "disabled." But for any number of reasons you might not feel as if you belong to that group at all.

> I never saw myself as disabled. I've always been able to do whatever I wanted and I was lucky in that I grew up in a small community so all the kids knew me and didn't really treat me any differently. Then I went to high school and there were people from all over. My friends got diluted in the crowds and all of a sudden I was different and it seemed like a bad thing. There was a boy who used a wheelchair and everyone thought we should be friends but I really stayed away from him. I didn't want anyone to think I was disabled like him. I never had a single date all through high school. I think that now that I know I'm disabled things have gotten easier.

Able-bodied people don't seem as scared of me because they don't have to pretend along with me that everything is exactly the same for me. I don't exactly have a date every Saturday night, but I have lots more, and I'm no longer scared to go out with someone who is disabled.

Things can get complicated, however, when you "qualify" for more than one "minority" identity. In addition to living with a disability or chronic illness, you may find yourself to be different from your peers in other ways. Friends who share one, but not all, of these identities may see this as *the* defining thing about you (so, to them, you are Muslim, or Protestant, first, and everything else is in the background). Some of us who have a minority sexual identity (like being gay, or bisexual) may find it particularly hard to disclose this identity to our families, who we may feel have had a lot to deal with related to our disabilities.

It took me a long time to admit to myself that I was gay. I just didn't want to have to deal with some other big thing in my life. I really didn't want to tell my parents. It has been hard for them bringing me up. It has sometimes been expensive for them, and I know they always worried about me. So, I didn't want to put them through another hard time. Also, I didn't think they would react very well. But then I fell in love and I wanted them to know that John wasn't just a good friend. So I told them that I was gay. They looked kind of stunned; I don't think they had a clue. Then my mother asked if I was seeing someone and I told her that I was in love with John. She started to cry and said that she had always worried that I wouldn't find someone to love who would know how terrific I am and she was glad I had. Now it was my turn to be stunned. My father has taken longer to come around to the whole thing, but he and John both love football, so it gives them something to talk about.

I volunteer at a disability organization. Some of the staff are in relationships and openly talk about them, but I don't feel included in this. No one knows I'm gay and I feel like the things that are important to me are never spoken about or ever mentioned. I wonder how many people who are gay who come to this center feel invisible?

It may get easier to integrate these various things into your image of yourself as you do it more. So, coming out as gay or lesbian may not seem like such a big deal when you already live with being obviously Latino, and very short, and on dialysis.

Who identifies us first can also have an impact on how comfortable we feel. If you live with a visible disability, it is an identity that you live with, whether you choose to or not. Others have decided that you have a disability, and likely informed you of it early in life. You didn't get to discover it or to choose how much of your identity it would be. Chances are it was made clear to you that this part of who you are was a limitation. By contrast, some families actively deny their child's disability, and that denial can also be a barrier to developing a positive identity that includes disability.

Being pushed to the edges of society because of being identified with a group is particularly hard for children, who often absorb the negative stereotypes of the group into their fledgling sense of who they are. It is important to think about the things we learned as children and the lessons we still carry with us. A positive interaction with friends, particularly in adolescence, can have a profound effect on developing a strong disabled identity. But as we buy into society's negative stereotypes of who we are, and have them constantly drummed into us, we may push ourselves beyond the limits to prove that we don't have a disability at all.

There is another way: Instead of accepting the ideas we receive about disability, we can choose to call ourselves "disabled" and embrace an identity that brings us power, confidence, and pride.

I don't think the idea of me being a sexual person has ever seriously crossed the minds of the people in my family. To them oftentimes I think I'm seen more like a kid than a women even though I am 22.

I've never felt particularly good about my looks or my sexuality/ sexiness. This is somewhat due to my mostly unsuccessful attempts at finding sexual partners. I'm getting better, but I ain't there yet! Sex is very important to me because I feel if people see me as a sexual person, they can truly accept me as a whole person.

I have always felt very positively about my body and my disability, which has contributed greatly to my sex-positive outlook, and vice versa. Being born with a disability, I've never felt I was "missing" something.

Coming Out as Disabled

For years I did a lot of political work on different issues. Then I became sick and, after trying different treatments, realized that I wasn't going to get better. I was in denial for a long time, in the hopes that things would change. They didn't. I really saw for the first time how people treat people with disabilities—

FINDING MYSELF

During my teen years I was sure that I would remain forever a virgin and despaired about myself. I would spend long hours looking at myself in the mirror convinced I was the ugliest thing ever to walk the planet. I contemplated killing myself and found it very difficult to enter parties or crowded rooms. I wore clothes that attempted to hide my body's missing parts and stood or sat in uncomfortable positions in a vain attempt to hide myself away.

It all changed when I joined a drama group at the age of seventeen and was embraced by a large group of young people who found me no weirder than they were. We all romped around together and I began to see that just because I found myself a total freak didn't mean that everyone did, or that they found freakdom as repulsive as I did. Since those times my image of myself has changed dramatically. In fact, those people launched me on a sexual career of some note and variety.

because that was how I was being treated. It was when I went to a conference with other women with disabilities that I realized that that was who I was, I was a woman living with a disability. It's still something that I'm getting used to in terms of how I see myself, but I feel less shame about getting what I need around accessibility and other things.

Coming out to ourselves as disabled can be an important step. The term *coming out* is usually reserved for people who are disclosing their sexual orientation or gender identity. For example, one might "come out" to family, friends, or coworkers as gay, lesbian, bisexual, transsexual/ transgendered, or intersexed.

The coming-out process is ordinarily something that happens after much reflection, soul searching, and personal exploration. It isn't the end of a journey but rather a point where you are finally accepting a particular identity for yourself and taking the risk of sharing that identity with the important people in your world. You are boldly stating "This is who I am, here and now, and it's not worth it for me to pretend or 'pass' anymore."

The ways that mainstream heterosexual society forces people to pass (that is, pretend to be heterosexual in public) are similar to the ways in which nondisabled society marginalizes the rest of us. Mainstream, nondisabled society has very specific rules for living with a disability.

> *After my accident my friends rallied around and visited me in the hospital, sent flowers, all that stuff. After a while though, I think they just wanted me to get on with things; it was like the disability was yesterday's news. I had done the disabled thing, now I could just stop being so boring and drop it. It wasn't like I talked about it all the time, or ignored their needs, but they just wanted it to be a total nonissue, which it could not be, mainly because of access issues and stuff.*

Coming out to others about your disability is, in part, about holding onto your right to take care of your own body and to maintain a close connection to it. Knowing when you get tired, realizing your limits, sensing when you're aroused by even the slightest physical cue—all are things that come with practice and are gifts that many others don't have. It's often assumed that disability creates a split between a person and their body because of the things they "lost." While this may happen to some, for many of us it's more true that learning to live with our disabilities brings us closer to our bodies.

How I feel about my body greatly affects my sexuality, and how I feel about my body is that it is great! I don't have a traditional body, but I have one that I am intimate with and one that has given me many moments of pleasure. I love my body! I think of myself as sexy and, therefore, others do too. I accent the positive and deemphasize the negative. The only time I've had trouble with my image of my body is when I have been unfortunate enough to allow a jerk to impact the way I feel about myself; however, I've always rebounded from those moments of embarrassment, though sometimes it's taken a while to build the ego back up. Chronic pain sometimes makes it hard to love my body because it makes me hurt, but even then, I can usually find nice ways to treat myself and make the body feel good.

Our society tends to define people as single issues. So our disabilities may become who we are to some people, rather than just one aspect of our lives. Everything about us is blamed on or credited to the disability. Sexually, this can have devastating consequences. We may be viewed as "heroic angels" who are too good to have sex, or as helpless victims, unable to do anything, *especially* have good sex.

My disability is very visible, but I can cover up the physical aspects of my disability sitting on a stool or a regular chair. The fact that I try to cover up my disability shows I do feel insecure about it. When I am on my knees people tend to put two and two together and I get praise for my "courage." But sometimes I just want to hear, "you have a nice smile, I like your body, and man can you party." Hearing about my courage and inspirational ability to meet my challenges becomes repetitive. I guess I want my disability to be set upon the back burner. But most of the time people seem to place it in the front.

I think my disability affects my self-esteem. I am about to graduate from college and possibly go to law school, which is something that many people whether or not they are disabled never do, but with all my achievements I still often feel as if other people don't really see those accomplishments because I am in a wheelchair.

It's all connected for me. I see myself as very sexual, and I think this makes me feel good about myself. My positive feelings about myself are pretty obvious, I think, so then other people see me as sexual and interesting and see my disability as part of that, and seeing all that in their attitudes, voice, actions makes me feel even sexier.

Taking Care of Ourselves

Our bodies are where self-esteem, desire, and sexuality come together. The more attention we pay to our needs, the better we are able to take care of ourselves. This can only have a positive impact on our sexuality.

When I was younger I really struggled with issues related to my disability, sexuality, and especially incontinence. I remember having a relationship with someone who had never been with someone with a disability—it was new for both of us. I was so fearful about telling him that occasionally when I get sexually excited, I pee. I felt badly about my body and that I couldn't always "control" it. He kept telling me it was okay and that I didn't need to worry. But it took a long time before I believed him. Years later I still catch myself struggling with this, even though I've had some successful relationships since then. You're just not sure how the other person is going to react even though you know that regardless of how they react, that fear still gets in the way.

I still run around some days, work too hard, get too upset at little things, all of which I know will lead to fatigue at the end of the day, which may trigger my pinched occipital nerve. Yet I persist. Until I'm willing to say that I need to take care of myself, that I can't do things either like I used to or like I see other people can, until I get to that point I just increase the chances that I'll have a flare-up of pain. It's okay to make a choice about that, to say to myself, "Well, I really want to do this and I want to do it all-out, and tomorrow I'll pay for it." But to do all that because I "forgot" that I shouldn't is a different thing.

How do we begin to challenge all the messages that are out there about living with a disability and having sex, having a sexuality, just believing that we are 'hot'? Through the process of individual change, we can challenge beliefs and have the opportunity to see things in different ways. Making a personal inventory of those messages we have put into our own belief system is a good way to start. The more we have a chance to see how "ableist" messages have personally affected us, the more we are able to nurture our own inner resources, strengths, and values. This is not to say that the following strategies are easy (we know this from our own experiences), but with practice there will be opportunities to shift how we think about ourselves.

Exercises

1. Make a list of all the things you could say after the words "I am...." Consider writing them down or saying them out loud. Some of these things will be individual characteristics, such as "I am a belly dancer" or "I am an avid reader." For those that are not related directly to sexuality, think about whether they have an impact on who you are as a sexual being.

   Make a second list of the groups you feel others have put you in. Think about the subtle and not so subtle ways other people's assumptions can impact the way you both think and feel about yourself. Then indicate which groups you feel you fit into, and add any that aren't on the list that you have made.

2. Make a list of the qualities that you value most about yourself and others. Now make a second list of qualities you wish you didn't have, and a third list of the things that people around you expect of

you. Think about people in your life whom you admire. In what ways do you think the qualities you have listed have contributed to their self-esteem?

3. Get in touch with the disability or chronic health-related organizations that are supposed to be serving your needs. It might be the local American Cancer Society chapter, or your nearest center for independent living. Most organizations have acknowledged that they can't address just one aspect of who you are and hope to effect real change or support. So call or write, get someone's attention. Ask them if they consider sexuality to be an important part of an individual's life. Do they think that there is a connection between how we feel about ourselves in general and how we feel about ourselves as sexual beings? If the answer is no, ask them why not. If the answer is maybe, or yes, ask them what the organization is doing to support people's right to explore that part of their lives. Do they have any books or films, do they offer any courses? They may conduct dozens of life skills courses on balancing a checkbook (which is admittedly important), but how many times have they given a course on how to meet someone if you want to date, or what to do if you just want to have sex with someone? You can take this exercise as far as you like. You're going to get plenty of silence on the other end; sometimes you'll get lectures from people obviously opposed to even speaking about sex. But occasionally you'll get someone who is genuinely interested, and thankful that you've called to raise the subject. The more people who do this, the closer to the surface the topic will get.

3

Sexual Anatomy and Sexual Response

*I get the feeling people think that because I am in
a chair there is just a blank space down there.*

Underlying much of what is written about disability and
sexuality is the idea of deficiency. These writings usually
tell us about what we won't feel, what we can't do, and
the ways we can make up for the fact that we aren't
getting the "real thing." Despite what people actually
experience, many of us still view sex as something that
is the same for everybody considered "normal," and
inferior for the rest of us. But every person needs to
discover what sex is for them—how it feels, and what
they respond to.

*Yeah, sex is definitely different since I got
injured. Now I use a wheelchair and I don't*

always get erections when I want. Things are slower in some ways, but when I do have the chance to have sex I really like it, and figure it's probably different than it would be if I wasn't in a wheelchair. Like, there are parts of my body now that are so sensitive to touch and I can't believe how easily I get turned on by having my nipples and ears touched. So I don't think of it as bad, just different.

Constructing a sexual blueprint that maps the places on your body where you have more or less sexual sensation, as well as what your body looks like (inside and out), its textures and rhythms—leads to a healthier sexuality. In this chapter we propose a radically different way to approach our sexual anatomy and response, departing from the ways most books write about it.

We almost wrote this chapter without any description of what most people's genitalia look like, intending to leave it to you to discover what *you* look like. But we found three problems with this. To start with, you may not be able to see or feel some (or any) parts of your body. Second, with no descriptions or pictures, you don't have the opportunity to put names to the sexual parts of your body. This can make it hard to communicate with sexual partners, as well as with people to whom you might turn for advice. Third, many kids with disabilities who have the usual sexual anatomy grow up thinking that there is something different and unusual about the way they look sexually, primarily because they have picked up on the societal message that they are not sexual beings and will never become so. It can be empowering to realize that you probably do have everything that your friends have "down there." People who have differences in their sexual anatomy may be surprised at how many similarities there are. Your body may be different, in how it looks, functions, or feels, from the usual way things are, but in this book we won't use terms like *normal* and *abnormal*.

Even though my penis looks very different than other guys, it works fine. I had several operations when I was a kid, to "fix" how it looked and so that I could pee better. There is some scar tissue from that where I don't have much feeling, but I don't notice that during sex. When I was younger, I would have given anything to look normal. I still don't use the urinal, but always go into a stall so no one can see me. But now that I have a girlfriend who doesn't mind how it looks, what's important is that she and I both get pleasure from it.

Your disability is part of who you are. Your chronic fatigue, mobility limitation, or lower body paralysis is as much a part of your sexual self as your enviable upper body muscles, sweet tush, gorgeous breasts, or graceful hands. Your body is the raw material you get to work with. You might as well get acquainted with the whole package.

Barriers to Understanding Our Bodies and Our Sexuality

Those of us who have been living with our disabilities from birth or childhood have had a lifetime to get to know our bodies, but may have missed out on basic sexual health education. People new to living with a disability may have to discover what this means sexually. People with progressive illnesses may have to constantly adapt to changes in sexual functioning. Also, people whose genitalia look fairly standard will have a different perspective from those whose genitalia don't.

In addition to the negative beliefs many of us heard while growing up (sex is dirty, only bad people touch themselves, pleasure is suspect), anyone who has had prolonged contact with the health care system as a child has had their body treated as if it is a foreign object—something to be cleaned, prodded, exposed, or hurt, something that is the property of the people in the system. We can overcome this childhood training and learn more about how we feel, what excites us, what makes us feel good.

Teens especially face a number of barriers as they work toward becoming sexually healthy adults. Medical appointments or hospitalizations may result in missing the few sex education classes that are given in early adolescence. Parents may assume that a child with a disability is not a sexual being, and the teen will pick up on that assumption and may come to believe it. Institutions and families may choose a prohibitive approach to risk taking, so teens are protected from risk and do not know how to judge levels of risk or how to protect themselves from harm in any way other than totally avoiding things that might be risky. A parent and a teen may both resist any separation from the other, whether emotional or physical, even though separation on some level is a key element in developing identity, exploring sexuality, and growing up.

Differences in the rate of physical development can also make things hard for teens. Some disabilities are associated with early puberty, and may lead to feelings of embarrassment or shame. Other teens experience late puberty, and get treated as if they are much younger than their age, being seen as nonsexual.

As adults, we face many barriers to exploring our bodies and sexual feelings, many of which result from issues of identity and self-esteem. One of the problems with addressing these concerns is that they usually take a backseat to more obvious, functional issues. So instead we might dwell on looking for partners, all the while ignoring the fact that we may have attached all our feelings of self worth to finding the partner in the first place. This is something everyone does, to some extent, regardless of disability. We don't need to "have it all figured out" before we go out and look for other people to be sexual with.

One other barrier exists, particularly for people whose bodies and genders don't fit within the narrow definitions of male and female. Those of us who identify as transsexual or who are intersexed can be frustrated by the fact that most discussions of sexual anatomy and response force us to choose one type of gender identity (they tell us that if you're a woman you'll feel *this* way, or if you're a man you'll feel *that* way). In parts of this chapter we fall into this trap ourselves, and while we avoid doing this as much as possible, the limits of language and space in this book meant that we haven't always succeeded.

Become Your Own Sex Expert

Despite all the myths you've grown up with and the barriers imposed on you, the good news is that you have limitless ways to explore your own body. No one else can figure out the best way for you to do this. We will make some suggestions and leave it to you to figure out how to make them work for you.

In general, people lack knowledge about sex. To varying degrees we are all ignorant of our sexual options, ignorant of sexual possibilities, and even ignorant about our own bodies. If you're nondisabled and you want to educate yourself, it isn't always easy to do, but at the very least you always have access to your own body, and sometimes privacy, too. By contrast, if living with your disability prevents you from having access to your whole body, you are often, quite literally, at the mercy of others. We don't just mean being able to masturbate, or put on a condom, or position yourself for sex with a partner. We also mean being able to see what your whole body looks like. It's hard to take control of your sexuality when you may not know the raw materials you're dealing with.

For some people it won't be feasible to see and touch all parts of their bodies. If you require twenty-four-hour assistance you may never have someone willing to hold a mirror to see what your clitoris looks like. You may not feel comfortable even asking for that help.

> My doctor said I should have a Pap smear, even though I've never had sex. He sent me to another doctor who has a hydraulic exam table. Even with that it took a lot of maneuvering to get me into position. Then she said, "My nurse can hold a mirror so you can see what I'm looking at and doing." I said, "Oh that's gross, I don't want to see that." But she told me it wasn't gross and that I should take a look. It was really cool.

In most standard sex manuals the advice is the same: Own your body. And in these books "owning" is usually defined by seeing. There are several obvious "ableist" assumptions here. We don't all experience reality through sight. Does this mean that we're just screwed (so to speak)? We'd say no. You have other ways to explore your body.

Getting Support

Now that we've made our arguments for all the reasons to become your own sex expert, there are some potential risks we want to mention. As with any form of self-discovery you run the risk of finding out stuff that is difficult to deal with along with stuff that is exciting and fun. Often memories are linked to sensations. We will smell something and a childhood episode will flood back. We are touched in a certain way and another memory arises. Without a stimulus, these memories can remain hidden for years. The exercises we mention throughout this chapter, and at the end of it, involve working with your body and getting more in touch with your body, which may trigger memories from the past, both pleasurable and traumatic.

What supports will you need to have in place in case you need to deal with things that come up during your experience? You may have overwhelming feelings that you don't know how to cope with. Do you have someone you can talk with about these strong feelings or memories? If you don't have a friend, family member, or caregiver with whom you can hash things out, or some other way that you work through difficult things in your life, you should consider getting the number of a crisis or help line. Phone lines are not accessible to everyone, but there may be other community or Internet resources, such as TTY machines available on some public pay phones. Some people also find it helps to listen to music or write when faced with tumultuous emotions.

You may be quite out of practice in thinking about your body as something worth getting in touch with. It's possible that part of this whole "getting in touch" thing means becoming more aware of physical or psychological pain. So take the time you need to decide if and when it's worth doing this.

We don't mean to make this seem scary or make it necessarily a big deal. But we speak from personal experience—support can be very important when doing any sort of self-discovery.

Sexual Anatomy

You may have heard sex educators speak of every part of your body being a potential sex organ. That's great news, don't you think? But it's one thing to say that and another to realize that potential. Here we will talk about various parts of the body and offer some tips on self-exploration. As with everything in this book, no one method will work for everyone, so feel free to tailor our suggestions to your needs. It would be silly to assume we're all the same and our paths to sexual discovery are the same, so take what seems to be helpful and leave the rest. First we will talk about some basic approaches and environmental factors you may want to be aware of or create.

Although for many people the most intense sexual feelings happen in the body parts we will describe below, much of the feeling of excitement and release comes from more general body feelings. When sexually aroused, we all have an increase in heart rate, breathing, body temperature, and blood pressure. Blood collects in various places, including the ears and lips. The skin gets flushed, sometimes especially on the chest and neck. All of these things intensify. If there is no orgasm, they gradually settle down. If an orgasm occurs, they resolve more quickly. The rapid fall in body temperature—as well as the pleasurable feelings of release and sexual satisfaction—often makes people fall asleep.

Breathing

You may be wondering why we begin our discussion of sexual anatomy with breathing. Although we may do it differently, breathing is something we all do, and we can all have some awareness of. What we propose is a way of using your breath to take a guided tour of your own anatomy.

There are many different schools of thought on breath awareness, and what we present here combines what we have learned from some of them. The majority of people reading this book can control their breathing to some extent. However, breathing may be difficult because of lung diseases, muscle weakness, heart disease, or problems with the nerves that make breathing happen automatically. Paying attention to the breath will not make any of these things worse; in fact it may help them. If you do not have control of your breathing and use a ventilator, you have probably already noticed that your vent rate can affect how you feel—more energized when the rate is higher, more relaxed when it is lower.

Breathing, like sex, can be both energizing and relaxing. One of the great unspoken benefits of sex play is the relaxing effect it has on most of us afterward. Sex is a great way to deal with insomnia (like nature's sleeping pill!). It is an excellent form of pain management, can help with spasms, and increases blood flow. Many of these benefits occur because of what happens to our breathing when we're having sex.

> *Because of my disability my parents are very protective. They always listened to make sure I was okay. I always felt I had to be really quiet when I would masturbate. When I first started having sex with my boyfriend, I was in the habit of being really quiet. I'd expend a lot of energy not making noise. Often I'd be holding my breath, without even realizing it. Then he said, "Don't you like this? You're all tense and you never make a sound." I realized I didn't need to hold myself back.*

We don't all breathe at the same rate, nor can we all do complicated Tantric breathing rituals (more on those in chapter 10).

Conscious breathing is probably the oldest known technique to bring your attention to your body. We breathe in mainly through the efforts of the diaphragm, a thin, domed muscle that stretches under the lungs. When the diaphragm flattens, it pulls down, making the pressure in the chest less than that in the atmosphere, so air flows in. We also have "accessory" muscles that can help us breathe in, though we don't use them as much. When the diaphragm relaxes, it goes back to its dome shape and air flows out of the body. Breathing in (inhalation) takes muscular effort, while breathing out (exhalation) is a result of relaxation. Air flows through the nose or mouth and into the trachea, a large tube that splits into two smaller tubes (bronchi) that take air into the lungs where

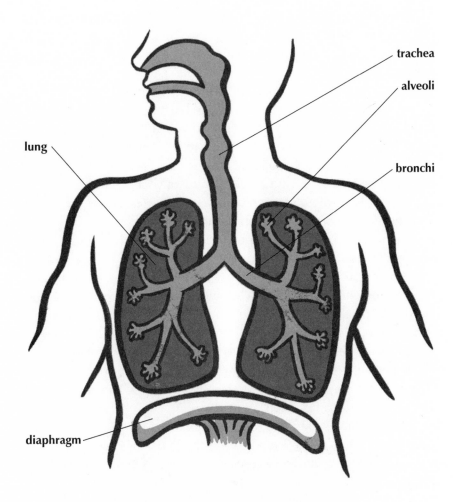

Illustration 1. Respiratory System

it ends up in little air sacs (alveoli). Oxygen from the sacs goes into the bloodstream, and waste products in the body, like carbon dioxide, go into the alveoli and then leave the body during exhalation. We breathe more heavily when we need more oxygen.

When practicing with the breath, it is always easier emotionally to play with the exhalation, as it is a relaxing breath. If you find yourself feeling distressed, concentrate on breathing out, and try to gradually lengthen your exhale.

Breathing is something our bodies usually do involuntarily. Most of us have at least some control over when to breathe, when to make noise (talking or otherwise), and when to exhale. We go through our days not using this control, instead just letting it happen. This is a good thing, in general. By breathing automatically, we free ourselves to do other things. But it can be helpful to learn to take control of your breath.

Find a place where you can be comfortable. Try different positions and find one in which you are minimally distracted by your body. You may want some cushions to prop you up. Your position should be as symmetrical as possible, so if you can't sit, it is better to lie on your back than on your side. Close your eyes if you wish. Breathe normally and observe your breath. Count the seconds it takes you to breathe out. Slowly extend the exhalation. How do you feel when it takes longer? What if you pause between breathing out and breathing in? Then do the same with inhale. Count the seconds your inhale takes and then extend it. Try holding your breath at the end of the inhale. Do you notice a change in the way any part of your body feels (toes, ears, anywhere)? This is enough for a first effort.

The next time you try this, do the same things and then experiment with sound. Most of the sounds we make (moaning, talking, singing, yelling) come from our vocal cords at the top of the trachea. We also make some quiet noises (like whispering) by moving air around the back of the throat, through either the nose or the mouth. What sounds can you make breathing through your nose, then your mouth? How soft a noise can you make? How loud? Do each of these things slowly and make mental notes on how they feel. Now do the same thing with your vocal cords, trying out kinds of sounds. The next time, start playing with your inhale and exhale again, then explore the differences with breathing through your nose or mouth. You can breathe in through one and out the other, then switch.

Now try to imagine that you are sending the breath to different parts of your body. You can imagine it flowing to your head, your fingers, your genitals, your toes—to any part of your body, whether or not you have feeling in that area.

Take a Tour

You don't need to be able to move or to control your movements to take a tour of your anatomy. If you are lying down with your eyes closed, no one will even know you are awake. All you have to do is devote some time to focusing on one part of your body through your thoughts and your breath. Try not to make this "one more thing that you are required to do in life." Stop whenever you need to. Even five minutes can be used productively.

Start by doing some of the breathing that we talked about earlier. Then choose a part of your body to focus on. It doesn't have to be a part that you identify as sexual. Pick an area that doesn't usually cause you pain, or, if you have pain all over, an area where the pain is less intense or frequent. As you begin to focus on this part of your body, thoughts may float into your head. You may remember things that have been said about that part of your body, or the way it has been touched in the past (pleasant, unpleasant, neutral). Either give yourself permission to think of these thoughts, or put them aside and return to your breathing and your focus.

Imagine that with each inhalation you are sending your breath to this part of your body. After a while, you will notice that you are perceiving this part differently—it might seem bigger than usual, or tingling. If it is a spot where you have no sensation, concentrate on what it looks like, or imagine a string that connects it to somewhere that you have sensation, and that as you are breathing in, the string tugs on the other part. If you imagine your breath has a color that you are sending to that part of the body, a warm color (red, yellow, or orange) may lead to a warm feeling in the area, and a cooler color (blue, green, lilac) might make it feel cooler.

If possible touch that part of your body, with your hand or with something hooked up to an assistive device (back-scratcher, feather duster, soft piece of cloth), or direct a partner to touch you there. You may be able to move that body part against a pillow, a book, the edge of something. If you are sitting in front of a fan or a window, pay attention to how the breeze feels. If you can use your hands, try different kinds of touch, firm and light; use fingertips or the palm of your hand; a dry or wet finger; circular or linear motions. You may be able to use your tongue to explore your lips, gums, and the roof of your mouth.

Pay attention to how these things feel (pleasurable, sexual, uncomfortable?) and also to what you are learning about how that part of your body is put together—what is its shape? Lumpy or smooth, hard or soft, ridged or flat?

We suggest you approach your whole body this way. Find things that work for you, whether they be sight, smell, touch, or feelings of different levels of heat in various body parts. *Don't* avoid the parts that you have learned to think of as ugly.

In the following sections we will describe the parts of your body usually thought of as sexual. We happen to think many more parts are sexual, but you don't need us to tell you what a finger is, or an ear. The parts of our bodies that have been labeled "sexual" have been much more mystified.

As you are exploring your body, you may notice that the edges of things may be more sensitive—like the skin surrounding your nostrils, the sides of your fingers, the borders of your armpits, the areas right next to where you have no sensation. In addition, some people find that areas where they have no sensation of touch may respond to more direct pressure.

Also remember that just because a part of your body gets touched a lot (like your head against a headrest) doesn't mean that you can't experience touch to that part of you in a very different and sexual way.

Breast/Nipples

Many women like to explore the sensations of having their breasts or nipples touched. Fewer men do so. For some heterosexual men, breasts are so strongly identified as feminine that the idea of having their breast or nipples played with stirs up concerns about their sexual orientation. (We promise that if you are a straight man and you want to find out if your breasts/nipples are sensitive, it won't make you gay!)

Our culture places tremendous emphasis on how breasts look, rather than how they feel. Although we want you to look at your breasts, with a mirror or by looking down at them, we suggest you focus more on how they feel. You may notice variation in skin sensations over different parts of your breasts, as well as between light and firm touch, licking, squeezing, or pinching.

The nipple is a bump right in the middle of the breast. It has a small opening for milk to come out of. The size and shape of nipples vary widely—some look like pencil erasers, others are flat. Nipples have vessels inside that fill up with blood when we become sexually excited or when we feel cold. This makes them hard, the same way a penis gets an erection. Many people, but not all, crave nipple stimulation. Some enjoy a light touch while others like to have their nipples sucked on, twisted, pinched, or pulled.

The darker area around your nipple is called the *areola*. It may have some bumps around the edge. The skin of your areola may feel different to the touch from the skin of the rest of your breasts.

Breasts, in both men and women, are a combination of fat and milk-producing tissues. Men have very little milk-producing tissue. Some medications may cause an increase in this tissue. Women who have been pregnant (especially those who have breastfed) may find that a bit of milk seeps out of their nipples when their breasts are played with.

Touch your nipples with a dry finger and then a wet one. What does it feel like to squeeze it or pull on it?

Vulva (Clitoris/Labia/Urethral Opening/Vaginal Opening)

We encourage any woman reading this to find a way to look at her vulva. You may be able to hold a mirror between your legs with one hand and spread your labia apart with your other hand and look. Many doctors who do pelvic exams have mirrors for patients to use and will provide a "guided tour" of the area.

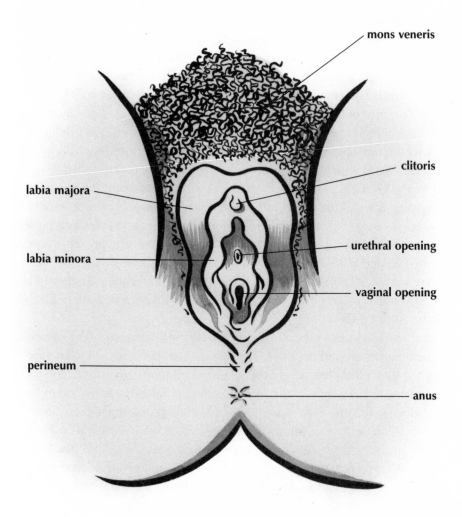

Illustration 2. Female Anatomy, External

Pubic hair often covers a triangular area. The top part is called the *mons veneris,* the lower parts are thick folds of skin called the *labia majora* (this just means "big lips" in Latin). The insides of the labia majora are usually pink and can be smooth or a bit ridged.

In between the labia majora is another set of skin folds called the *labia minora* ("little lips"). These are much thinner and more flexible than the labia majora and they have more blood vessels and nerve endings. When a woman is sexually excited the labia turn a darker color and may get thicker.

These lips come together at the top into a little hood that covers the *clitoris*. The external part of the clitoris (and that until recently was thought to be the whole thing) sits under the top of the labia minora. This is the tip of the clitoris, which is often less than an inch long but can be longer. It is made mainly of erectile tissue, spongy bodies that can fill up with blood, making it firmer and larger. Some people have more sensation in one part of the clitoris. If you are using your fingers to explore this area, start gently and use a lubricated finger. What you won't be able to directly feel or see is that the clitoris extends into the body and down in two roots to either side of the vagina. All of this can swell when sexually stimulated.

When a woman becomes sexually stimulated her clitoris becomes hard. Some women describe a throbbing feeling, while others say that as the clitoris becomes erect it gets more sensitive to touch. As it gets bigger, it may poke out from under its hood. Just before orgasm, the clitoris may pull back further under the hood. During orgasm the clitoris may pulsate or twitch.

Erectile tissue also surrounds the *urethral opening* (the hole women pee out of). To the sides of the vaginal opening are the *greater vestibular glands* (Bartholin's glands), which make a small amount of lubricating fluid. You won't be able to see these glands and usually they can't be felt.

Urethral Sponge (G-Spot)

A number of glands surround the *urethra* between the bladder and the urethral opening. Fluid is produced in these glands and may be released into the urethra during orgasm. This clear fluid then squirts out of the urethra. Some women make enough fluid that they notice it, even to the extent that it is similar to ejaculation in men. Many also find that they have a sensitive spot inside the vaginal opening that can be stimulated

LOOKING FOR YOUR G-SPOT

If you want to find for your G-spot here are a few steps that might work for you.

First, get turned on. It is easier to find your G-spot if you are already aroused because, as with most people, when you get turned on your G-spot becomes full of fluid and is a little bigger and firmer to the touch. Next, get into a position that makes it easiest for you or a partner to put a finger (a sex toy will work just as well) in your vagina and feel toward the front wall, as if you are touching toward your belly button. The G-spot is less than two inches inside your vagina and toward your belly. If you are using a toy it's best to get something that is either curved specifically for G-spot stimulation, or that is firm and won't bend when you insert it. If you are using a finger, when you insert it make a sort of "come hither" motion with your finger (curving it). The G-spot feels like a small, firmer spot; people say it's anywhere from the size of a dime to a quarter. You may actually feel the tissue itself, or you may feel the effects of it being stimulated.

and that then swells and gives a different sensation during orgasm. This area, on the front of the vaginal wall, is called the *G-spot* (after Ernst Grafenberg, who described it in 1950). "Finding" your G-spot isn't always easy or even possible. Even if you have full use of your arms, hands, and legs, sticking a couple of fingers into your vagina and past the pubic bone might require longer fingers or more flexible hips than most of us have. Still, sticking your fingers into your vagina and feeling around can be highly instructive even if you don't encounter your G-spot. Keep in mind, the G-spot is not some magical ticket to mind-blowing orgasms. Rather, it's just another part of your body that may or may not feel good when stimulated. If you can't reach, a dildo, an insertable vibrator, or a willing partner can help.

Vagina/Cervix/Uterus

The *vagina* is a tube that is lined with membranes similar to those in the mouth; unlike the mouth, it tends to be ridged or bumpy. Most of the nerve cells in the vagina are located in the outer third. The vagina is usually collapsed, with little space between the walls. It's self-lubricating and is typically a little wet with fluids. When sexually aroused

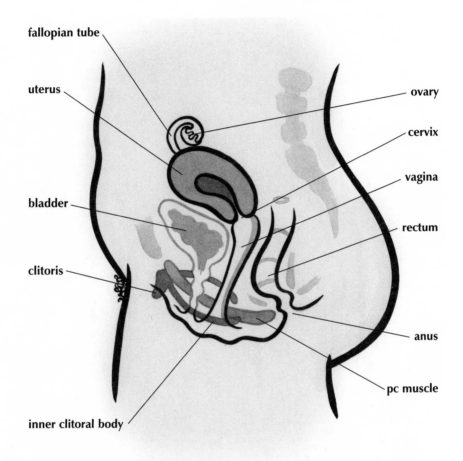

Illustration 3. Female Anatomy, Internal

many women find the lubricating fluids increase. Stimulation also enlarges the vagina. At the top of the vagina lies the *cervix,* which is also the bottom part of the *uterus.* Unlike the vagina, the cervix has many nerve cells. The cervix and uterus both swell during sexual excitement. The opening in the cervix becomes bigger and stays open for up to half an hour after orgasm.

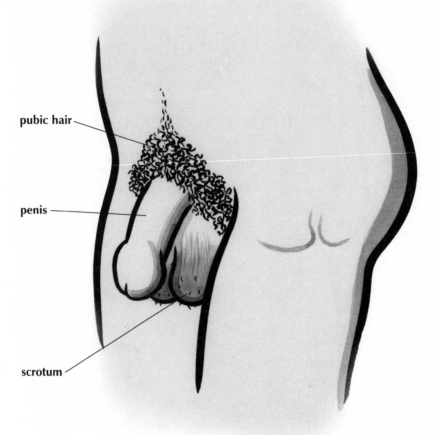

pubic hair

penis

scrotum

Illustration 4. Male Anatomy, External

Penis/Scrotum/Urethra

The *penis* has neither bone nor muscle in it. But at its very base it does have a few muscles (called *bulbar muscles*). The shaft of the penis is made up of two cylinders of spongy, erectile tissue. This tissue fills up with blood during sexual excitement, causing the penis to get bigger and harder, which is what an erection amounts to: blood-swollen tissue. A third cylinder on the underside of the shaft surrounds the *urethra*, the tube that carries both urine and ejaculate out of the body. Some men find having their urethra stimulated very pleasurable, while others find it uncomfortable. This stimulation may be intentional as a form of sex play or may be a side effect of having a catheter removed. The urethral opening is in the head of the penis, or *glans.* The underside of the glans, called the *frenulum,* contains the largest concentration of nerve endings. Men with genital sensation often find this area responds to stimulation the most intensely. Other areas along the shaft of the penis may also be highly sensitive to touch.

Some men are "uncut," while others are "cut," meaning that they were circumcised (their foreskin has been removed). The *foreskin* is a piece of skin that at birth covers the head of the penis and that can be pulled back to urinate, or pulled back and forth by pleasurable friction during sex. One of the main functions of the foreskin is to protect the head of the penis. Some parents have their male infants circumcised for a variety of reasons, medical, cultural, and religious.

At the base of the penis is the *scrotum,* a fleshy sac that holds the *testicles* outside the body. While this area can be very sensitive to pain, many men enjoy both the feel and the look of having their scrotum pulled down or squeezed (in fact several toys let men do just this, which we cover in chapter 9). The main function of the scrotum is to protect the testicles from injury and also to regulate their temperature, important for sperm production. During sexual arousal, the scrotum gets thicker and the testicles move up closer to the body.

Perineum

In women, the *perineum* lies between the vaginal opening and the anus, while in men it lies between scrotum and anus. Some men get pain in this area during arousal, in which case a gentle massage of the perineum can make the difference between a pleasant and a painful sexual experience. One reason for this might be that when a man's perineum is massaged, the prostate gland is also gently pressured. Rubbing this area is also sometimes called doing an external prostate massage. Other men, and women, enjoy having this area stimulated.

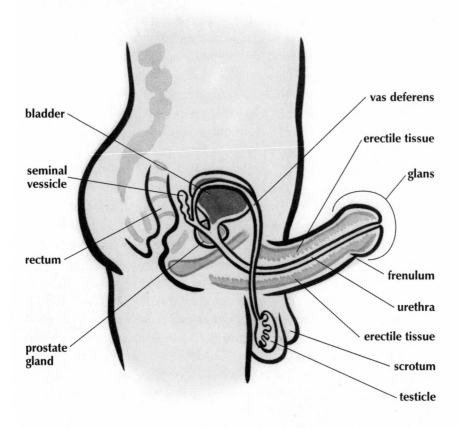

Illustration 5. Male Anatomy, Internal

Ass/Anus (and Prostate for Men)

In case you hadn't noticed, the ass has a great shape for being cupped in someone's hands. It also often comes in contact with other surfaces, and if you have feeling in that area but can't reach it with your hands, you can try sitting on textured surfaces (silk, fake fur, wood...) and rubbing back and forth. If you can reach the area, you can also explore the crack between the ass cheeks.

One of our favorite sex educators, Dr. Carol Queen, says the thing she loves about assholes is that everybody has one! This is almost always true, even if some of us have some differences in how they look or feel, or whether we can use them for elimination. People who don't have sensation around their penis, labia, clitoris, and other parts may well have lots of sensation around or in the anus, which can be a wellspring of sexual feelings.

The *anus* and *rectum* form the last part of the *gastrointestinal (GI) tract*. The very strong muscle of the *anal sphincter* surrounds the rectum. The anal opening (or anus) leads to the rectum, which curves to meet the *sigmoid,* which in turn leads to the *colon* and *intestines*. The delicate rectal tissue is made of blood vessels, nerves, and smooth muscle and is lined with cells that are in the same family as skin cells. The rectum, unlike the vagina, has no natural lubrication; like the vagina, it can expand, just not as much. The outside of the anus has lots of nerve endings around it. Many people with no genital sensation still are quite sensitive around their anus, thus this area can provide intense pleasure.

I can tell you it took me a while to get comfortable with it, and it's not like I like anything really big up there, but I find the area around my bum still has a lot of sensation, and I never knew before that it could feel so good. Now we've tried toys and other things and it's really a whole other feeling.

Internally, the other significant sexual part of the body for men is the *prostate gland*. The prostate can be felt through the rectum, toward the front of the body. It produces most of the fluid in ejaculate. Some men like to have their prostate directly stimulated with a finger, toy, or penis. As a result of medical conditions or medications, some men will have enlarged prostates that can be a source of pain or discomfort, yet for others it is a marvelous sex organ.

Sexual Response

When I was thirteen, the only time I knew I would be alone was on Sunday afternoon. My sister went to a church youth group, my father got together with a group of friends, and my mother would cook a huge Sunday dinner. I'd be in my room doing "homework." I'd masturbate as the house filled with the smells of my mother's cooking. Even now, when I smell a roast in the oven, I get a hard-on. I guess I'll never be a vegetarian.

Sexual response is a broad term referring to reactions to stimulation that you experience as sexual. You may respond to a touch from a partner, rain hitting your face, an arousing thought you have just before you go to bed, a sexually charged scene in a film you're watching, even an interview with a sex educator (or sex worker) on the radio. In short, you may respond to something not intended to be sexual.

Sexual response is, to our misfortune, considered the cornerstone of "true" sexuality in our culture. Whether or not you are responding in the right way, with enough oomph, often enough, and to the right sort of person (god forbid you sexually respond to someone of the same sex, or much older than you, or...well, the list goes on) is a topic of a seemingly endless stream of self-help books, fashion magazine articles, and radio call-in shows. Great research is being done by people like Beverley Whipple, who are taking the time to discover the different ways we all respond to sexual stimuli. (Whipple has been doing work inclusive of people with disabilities for years. She's also one of the initial documenters of the famed G-spot.) The problem is that most of us confuse sexual response with sexual feelings and sexual pleasure. Sexual response is something that researchers try to measure in a somewhat objective way. But having sexual feelings, and feeling pleasure, is best defined subjectively by the individual caught up in the moment.

We distinguish between sexual response and sexual feelings because if your sexual response doesn't seem to match up "like it's supposed to," if you skip a stage, or if you don't seem to experience anything that's recognizable by the standard definition, it's assumed you are missing something. If you lack a classical sexual response you're usually branded someone who lacks sexual feelings, or someone who may be unable to feel sexual pleasure. But this is not necessarily the case. Below you'll find some very basic information about how doctors and researchers have characterized sexual response, along with some suggestions on using these definitions for your own exploration. You'll also find information on ways that living with a disability or chronic illness can affect sexual response. But we want to remind you again that just because something affects your sexual response, it doesn't necessarily also affect your ability to feel pleasure or to have sexual feelings.

As with most of the other accepted terminology around sexuality, the words we have for sexual response don't always jibe with real people's experience. If you live with chronic pain, the relationship between your desire and arousal will be something incomprehensible to a person who has never experienced such severe pain. If you live with post-traumatic stress disorder (PTSD) and tend to dissociate during sex play, your "response cycle" will likely be different—and that may be a healthy adaptation to your experience. (Chapter 13 will give more details about this.) So before we tell you how professionals explain sexual response, we want you to consider the following questions as a way of looking at your *own* sexual response.

How Do *You* Define a Sexual Feeling?

I was pretty good friends with my male coworker and I remember one evening having to work with him on a deadline. We were sitting close to each other looking at some materials. As he got up from the table his foot caught on my crutch and he stumbled forward. He caught his balance before falling on me (which I wouldn't have minded) and brushed his hand on my shoulder. For the first time I felt this tingle in my stomach, and my crotch was throbbing. I remember my leg spasming under the table. I was sure he could tell. Later when I went to the bathroom I checked my panties and they were soaked. I was surprised by my reaction as I never felt that way toward him before. I fantasized a lot about him later that night and played with myself before falling asleep—I had a great night's sleep.

A lot of us think that sexual response is something that happens in a bed, with a partner, and probably involves some sort of enormous release. This can happen, but it is only one of many ways to feel sexually and respond sexually. Listening to music, having your hair brushed, gazing into someone's eyes without fear can all be incredibly sexual moments. What would you include on your list? Think about the last time you were aroused, whether you expected it or not, whether you thought it was "appropriate" or not. That was a sexual moment, and you had a real sexual response.

What Started It Off?

I think my parents were pretty uncomfortable with talking to me about sex because they didn't want me to have expectations; however, my body had other ideas. I was thirteen and was in school and that was the first time I got a boner. I didn't know what it was. There was this pretty girl coming down the hall toward me. I was trying to look really cool and say "hi." As I was wheeling away from her I looked down and saw this huge bulge in my pants. I didn't know what to do. I don't have a lot of feeling in my legs and so sometimes I get a hard-on without knowing it...even today. It can be embarrassing so I keep my book bag on my lap just in case. Other times, it can be a great icebreaker when meeting someone new...only if she's got a good sense of humor.

The last time you felt sexy/aroused, what triggered it? Was it something external—a smell, noise, taste, or sound? Was it from the touch of another person, or something brushing against you? Was it from your own touch (which is also external, in a way)? Or was it triggered by something internal like a thought, a memory, or a dream?

What Does It Feel Like?

It surprised me when I realized [after my accident] that I could still get turned on. Since I don't have any feeling down there, I had never noticed that when I'm excited I get this fluttery feeling in my chest. It's not new, I just never paid attention to it before.

We can throw the term *sexual response* around; we can talk about skin flushes, increased heart rates, erectile tissue, and on and on, but more important than the physiological process is your interpretation of it. How do *you* experience feeling turned on? Do you feel your heart race, does a part of you tingle, does it get harder to communicate verbally, is it always pleasurable? (Sexual response doesn't always feel good and doesn't always come as a result of things we are enjoying.) Pay attention to your own sensations and thoughts, and see if you can find your own descriptions for these feelings. There are as many ways to feel a sexual response as there are things to turn us on in the first place. You won't always respond the same way, even if it's to exactly the same sort of stimulation.

What does this feeling make you want to do, think, or say? Do you want to have more of this feeling? Less? Feeling turned on might make you want to go out and talk to people, have sex with a partner, or stay home and touch yourself. It may make you happy, sad, angry, frustrated, or confused. These feelings are a crucial part of your sexual response.

Don't worry about whether your desires seem realistic to you. Trying to anticipate obstacles can get seriously unsexy, so for now just fantasize what you would like to do, and later you can decide how to deal with the barriers—or the opportunities!

Can You Distinguish Between Your Thoughts and Your Sensations?

Check out what's happening in your physical sensations and in your thoughts. Do feelings of being turned on lead you to fantasize about specific possibilities? Do your thoughts make you feel sexier? Or not sexy at all? Invariably sensation and thought interact and influence each other, but as with everything else, the goal is to learn more about what precisely happens for *you* when you're turned on. Are there signs you can read in your body that show you are responding physically to the pleasure you are experiencing? Are there specific thoughts that trigger responses in your body? In the same way that people report effects of being turned on in their body (for example, feeling more relaxed, experiencing less pain), people also describe changes in their thoughts (fewer negative thoughts, even less anxiety).

How Do You Know When It's Over?

Since I became paralyzed in both legs I have noticed that I have varying kinds of orgasms, depending upon the situation. For example, when I play with myself and rub my clit a certain way my orgasms are much more intense. Sometimes my leg will go into spasm and my crotch feels tingly. But when I am with my lover, I find that it is more difficult to have an orgasm even if he is doing everything right. I think it is because I rely on the sensation of my fingertips on my clit and lips and I am able to change how hard I press or how fast I rub based on how my clit feels on my fingertips. Sometimes, this is hard to explain to a lover because I am not always able to communicate clearly when I am feeling more sexually aroused. Eventually I do have an orgasm, and though they are satisfying, they are not as physically intense. I realize how it might be helpful for my lover to know what it is that I feel when I am masturbating so he knows what he may need to change or do differently.

In our view, too much is made of the finale of a sexual response. It's almost as if without a "proper" ending (which the experts always consider to be an orgasm) the experience somehow isn't valid. We think orgasms are great—for the bliss they provide as well as other benefits. Orgasms are a fine natural sleeping pill, and the least invasive form of pain management around. Many people who experience muscle spasms find the number of spasms reduced after orgasm. Yet all sorts of sex play can result in the pain reducing, spasm reducing, emotionally grounding effects people report from orgasms.

We don't all experience orgasms as described in sex guides and erotic films. Many of us get off on sex play without reaching orgasm. You may even be experiencing an orgasm and not know it because you're too busy expecting it to feel like something else—either something you experienced before, or something you've heard so much about.

All of us have experienced a sense of alienation from our bodies and our sexual response. We all need to allow ourselves our sexual thoughts, sensations, and feelings with as few pressures as possible. For now we suggest that you give yourself permission to consider *anything at all* to be the proper end of a sexual experience. It may be occurring when you get tired, or bored, or cramp up, or have to go to work. Or it could be those fabulous multiple orgasms accompanied by gushing ejaculation. Just don't spend all your sexual energy worrying about how it will end.

Sexual Response Cycles

Masters and Johnson were two sex researchers who did pioneering work in the area of human sexuality by actually measuring the body responses of people having sex in a laboratory setting. From this research Masters and Johnson developed a model of sexual response in which they divided sexual response into four stages: excitement, plateau, orgasm, and resolution. To each of these stages Masters and Johnson assigned physiological responses, such as erection as a response to arousal.

Another researcher, Helen Singer Kaplan, changed their model somewhat by adding desire to the conception of sexual response, and suggested only three stages: desire, excitement, and orgasm.

We don't see these stages as particularly useful. If you're one of those people who really gets off on research and science, check out any of the books in the Sexuality: Disability-Specific Resources section of chapter 14 for more detailed information. We do think that over time you will come to recognize your own sexual response: the signals your body gives you that it wants more of one thing and less of something else.

Arousal

Researchers have found certain common physical effects of getting turned on; these include faster heart rate, heightened muscle tension, increased blood flow, greater body warmth, the production of lubrication, swelling of the clitoris and vaginal lips in women's bodies, penile erections in men's bodies, nipple erections in both men and women, as well as increased sensitivity to stimulation and reduced sensitivity to pain.

Lubrication in women and erections in men can be stimulated in either (or both) of two ways. Our thoughts or memories can send a signal through the spinal cord to the genitalia, causing these signs of arousal. The other way is a reflex—a cycle of nerve stimulation that originates lower than the brain. Many men wake up in the morning with an erection, called a reflex erection. The signals for these come from the lower (sacral) area of the spinal cord. A person who has no sensation in their genital area still has nerves there that are connected to the spinal cord, so they can still have these signs of arousal. Genital stimulation can cause reflex lubrication or erection even when the person isn't aroused, and even if they don't want to have sex.

We recommend you try to pay attention to what it's like to get turned on both in your body and thoughts without putting physiological labels on the experience.

Erections

Getting an erection is something that both men *and* women may experience. As we said in the anatomy section, a number of body parts have erectile tissue in them—tissues that fill up with blood that is then trapped, making the area swell and become firm. This happens most obviously in the penis, but also in the clitoris, nipples, and earlobes. Erections carry an enormous social and personal meaning, particularly in men. Getting and keeping hard-ons, and having an orgasm through ejaculation, are a potent (pun intended) symbol of masculinity. A man might have difficulty, or be unable to get or maintain an erection because of reduced blood supply, changes in nerve stimulation, depression, or medications.

Ejaculation

For most men ejaculation and orgasm are synonymous, even though they are two distinct processes and experiences. This is better illustrated when we talk about women ejaculating. Despite some remaining controversy among researchers, most people who work in the area of sexual health education acknowledge that women have the capacity to ejaculate. (See our section earlier in this chapter on the G-spot.) While many women who ejaculate find it pleasurable, we would hate to see it become something else that people feel they must achieve sexually. There is already enough pressure around sex.

For women who live with incontinence, ejaculation (which often results from stimulation of the G-spot) may cause some distress. When women ejaculate, it looks, feels, and sometimes even smells a little like urine. But it's not. In fact, even if you live with incontinence, at times you may think you've peed, when in fact you ejaculated. Fear of being incontinent during sex keeps many people away from sex, while others have sex but get so preoccupied with worry about incontinence that pleasure is the furthest thing from their minds. Many manage to work through their initial fear (usually with a few peeing moments along the way) and discover that it is not the end of the world and does not have to "destroy the moment." We do what we can to lessen the chance of peeing during sex (such as not drinking coffee or tea or alcohol when we are planning or hoping to have sex, not drinking anything in the hour before, and peeing right before we have sex). None of these things will, however, prevent ejaculation. If we have only negative associations about fluid involuntarily coming out of our bodies, it may be hard to experience what some women call the "joy of squirting." On the other hand, knowing that ejaculation is possible gives an opportunity to think in a whole new way about getting all wet during sex. If there is the possibility of shooting some fluid during sex (whether pee or ejaculation), it's happening because we were in the throes of pleasure—which is surely a good thing. We're not trying to be glib about incontinence issues, but do want to point out how discovering parts of our sexuality that we're not usually told about can give us the chance to change the way we think about things. This is especially important when our thinking is so guided by nondisabled cultural norms.

Men are often unaware that they can have orgasms without ejaculating (and can ejaculate without orgasm), because these two things usually happen so close together as to be indistinguishable. Some men experience a type of orgasm called *dry orgasm* or *retrograde ejaculation*. When this happens a man will experience an orgasm but no ejaculate will come out. Usually this is because the ejaculate is emptied backward and flows into the bladder. This condition is not dangerous. Most men with dry orgasm claim that the sensation during orgasm is unchanged. In chapter 10 on Tantric sex we will share with you some exercises on learning to distinguish these two processes and to achieve orgasm without ejaculation. One thing that appears to be a biological reality is that after ejaculating there is a short period of time when ejaculating again is impossible. There is no evidence to suggest that continuing to experience sexual pleasure and even orgasm is impossible following ejaculation. Again, ejaculation is just one of many things that happen during sex—and part of finding a sexuality that feels right is choosing what to do, in what order, and when.

Orgasm

Orgasms come in all different shapes, sizes, colors, and textures. In our survey, people used all sorts of words to describe orgasms—everything from "wonderful" and "releasing," to "spiritual" and "mind-altering," to "painful" and "confusing." Orgasm is such a subjective experience that when we start to define it, it can seem as if there's a right way and wrong way to have one. There isn't.

You may never have had an orgasm and would like to experience them. People have told us that their doctor said they would never experience an orgasm, only to have one (or many) later in their lives. So it *is* possible.

Mitch Tepper, the founder of sexualhealth.com and a sexuality educator and researcher, has written extensively about orgasm. He writes both as a professional and a man living with a spinal cord injury. In reviewing the research on spinal cord injury (SCI), Tepper writes:

> About half of spinal cord injury survivors can experience orgasm and this ability is not strongly related to the level or completeness of injury. Some of us, for that matter, find sex even better than before injury. There is growing evidence that sexual knowledge, sexual self-esteem, and time since injury are related to the ability to experience sexual pleasure and orgasm. It seems that knowledge is power, power fuels self-esteem, and self-esteem opens the door to sexual pleasure.
>
> Orgasmic sex requires tuning in to our sensations—in the moment—and forgetting about quad bellies, atrophy, catheters, and making embarrassing sounds. It means not worrying about performing up to some imagined standard. And it means forgetting what we learned in the past about what is and isn't pleasurable.

The basic process of orgasm starts with a buildup of excitement through sexual interest and arousal. The body goes through changes, including increased heart rate, blood pressure, body temperature, and muscle tone, as well as physical changes like the testicles increasing in size and the vagina expanding. With orgasm comes a release that is associated with muscular contractions. Immediately following an orgasm we all have a period (called a refractory period) when we will not experience another orgasm. For some people this period is short, perhaps only minutes long, while for others it can be hours.

Multiple orgasms are a series of orgasms one after another. Reports suggest that women have a much shorter refractory period and, if they continue to receive stimulation, can experience more than one orgasm in a row. More recently it has been suggested that men too can experience multiple orgasms by learning to have nonejaculatory orgasms. Some women seem to roll from orgasm to orgasm quite rapidly.

How Do You Define Orgasm, Anyway?

It's important to remember that orgasm has been defined by nondisabled people observing the sexual behavior of other nondisabled people. So we can't expect to see much of our experience in the literature (whether it's a self-help book or a medical journal). People have chosen to distinguish orgasms in different ways.

Some people define orgasms based on what they feel like. Sex educator and author Betty Dodson distinguishes what she calls "tension orgasms," which are the result of tensing your body up during arousal and climax, from "relaxation orgasms," which come from a longer and slower buildup of excitement and pleasure.

Another way to distinguish orgasms is based on where we feel them and how we get them. Some women report that orgasms from clitoral stimulation feel different than orgasms through penetration (it is worth noting that not many women have orgasms through penetration alone, although some research suggests that women with complete spinal cord injuries may be experiencing these orgasms for a reason; see below).

These orgasms from penetration are also sometimes called "G-spot orgasms" because it is thought that they are the result of stimulation of the G-spot through penetration. Another type of orgasm occurs from fantasy alone. Some women with spinal cord injuries are able to have orgasmic response in their bodies without any form of physical stimulation. While this is probably not common, it is important to be aware of the possibility.

Several recent studies, in fact, have documented that some people with severe neurological impairment, including complete spinal cord injury, can experience orgasm. One team of researchers proposes the existence of a nerve pathway bypassing the spinal cord and accounting for women with complete spinal cord injuries experiencing orgasm through penetration (to be specific, induced through cervical stimulation). These reports dispel the myth that only certain kinds of nondisabled people can experience orgasm and that everyone else should just give up. The reality is that some of us won't be able to experience an orgasm, and some of us may choose not to experience them. But we ought not be told what is and isn't within our sexual sphere.

Many people report experiencing multiple orgasms, either as a series of orgasms in rapid succession or a series of mild orgasms building up toward a really powerful orgasm. Yet another type of orgasm people report is sometimes called a "whole body" orgasm or "extended" orgasm. When people describe these kinds of orgasms, they don't focus on genital muscular contractions or one particular part of their bodies.

> The first time I had what I would call a "whole body" orgasm it was as if the sex had lit a fire in my body and even though we were finished fucking I was still burning, but in a good way. The kind of orgasm I usually feel only in my hips and head was running up and down my body and it was like waves rolling over me. I was way more relaxed after that experience than I usually am after sex, and I know the relaxing effects lasted a lot longer also.

Living with a disability or chronic illness can impact our experience of orgasm in all sorts of ways. For many of us (regardless of disability), orgasm doesn't come "naturally." Not having orgasms can result from difficulties at any stage of the sexual process. It can relate as much to how you feel about your body as to the actual sensation you have in your clitoris or penis. If you're having difficulty experiencing orgasm it may also be related to medications (a side effect doctors often forget to mention). You owe it to yourself to find out.

Kegel Exercises

Many people have discovered the orgasm-enhancing benefits of exercising their pelvic muscles, particularly the pubococcygeal (PC) muscle, a sling that provides support for the genital area and is the main muscle we tighten when we want to stop the flow of our urine. Kegel exercises increase blood flow to the genitals and can restore vaginal muscle tone that has been lost. They heighten our awareness of the entire genital area. Positive sexual effects can include stronger orgasms as well as increased control over ejaculation. Many people who have incontinence when they cough, sneeze, or laugh can gain control over it using these exercises.

Kegel exercises involve squeezing the PC muscle. To find the PC muscle, try to stop the flow of urine while you are peeing. (You might not be able to feel your PC muscle the first time you try.) Tighten the PC

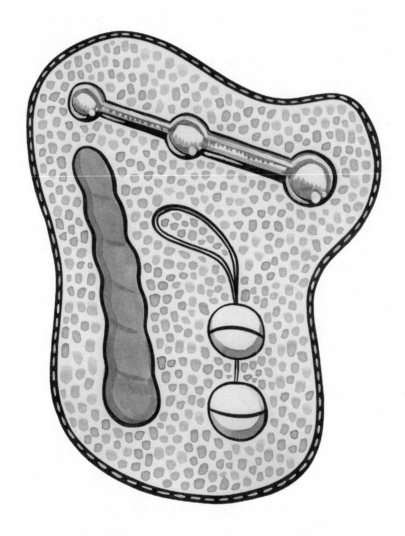

Illustration 6. Products to Use for Kegel Exercises

muscle and hold it for a few seconds, and then release. You can do this anywhere—on the bus, in a meeting (imagine the possibilities!), or lying down. If you can work up to squeezing for ten seconds, try this: Squeeze and hold for ten seconds and then release. Do this ten times and then stop. If you can repeat these exercises three times a day that's great, but just do as much as you can.

Another kind of squeezing exercise is to tense up your PC muscle and release as quickly as you can. Again squeeze and release quickly for a thirty-second workout. Do this several times a day. Eventually you will feel more control, and the feeling of tightening and releasing will become more defined.

Resistance Kegels involve "pulling up" or sucking in the muscles and then pushing out or bearing down. This is easier for women to do with something inserted in the vagina that they can try to draw in or push out. Men can imagine trying to draw their testicles up nearer to their body when "pulling up."

Kegel devices can make the exercises easier for women, but they aren't necessary. Most of these toys are cylindrical with a series of different-size, ball-shaped grooves in them. Women insert the ball into their vagina and then squeeze down on the ball itself. Or they can insert the toy a bit and then pull it out gently while trying to hold it in with their muscles.

Things to Consider About Your Own Sexual Response

It takes energy to feel sexual and to explore our sexuality. When we aren't interested in sex (professionals call this "reduced libido"), it may be that we simply lack the energy to feel sexual. Still, we remain sexual beings even when our interest or energy is low. A variety of other factors, both internal and external, may influence our level of sexual energy and interest, although they may not necessarily affect our experience of sexual pleasure.

Pain

What I hate is that sex is supposed to be something you just throw yourself into, but I have to plan almost every second of it to make sure that I don't end up in a position that makes my pain worse. Even when I stick with what I think are safe positions, I can still get

*pain from it. I masturbate in the bathtub. There isn't the same pres-
sure on my body and I can just float away on the experience. But
unless I find a rich lover who has a swimming pool, I don't think I
can translate this into a sexual experience with someone else.*

Pain can take over both our bodies and our lives, making it hard to focus
on anything else. Those of us living with chronic and debilitating pain
think ridiculous the very idea that we can experience an idyllic moment
of physical pleasure. We can find it hard to understand the often patron-
izing self-help language that encourages us to "embrace" our bodies,
"open ourselves up" to experience. Pain can have an impact every step
of the way along the sexual response continuum. In some obvious ways
it can dampen our ability to feel sexual pleasure, and our energy to do the
work involved. It can also suppress our motivation. When any amount of
energy results in some pain, even desire can end up being something
worth avoiding. On the other hand, recent studies show distraction is an
important tool in dealing with pain, and if we can allow ourselves to get
to the point of sexual pleasure, it can be a powerful tool for pain relief.

Since we are clever in finding ways to avoid or minimize pain with
all our other activities, we can apply these to sex play as well. If ecstasy
turns into agony after a minute of writhing your hips during sex, it may
help to use different muscles, or toys, or positions.

Fatigue

*If I go to a dance, when it is over I know lots of my friends are going
to have sex. But I have spent the afternoon in bed storing up
energy just to be able to dance for part of the time. I'm dead by
the end. So for me the choice is, have sex or go to the dance. I hate
this because I don't want every date to be just one or the other.
And, like, I'm supposed to say to my boyfriend, "Let's have sex
instead of going out"? I guess he could go to the dance alone afterward while I sleep.*

Fatigue is part of many chronic conditions and can also be caused by a
condition that requires a large expenditure of energy just to attend to

daily tasks. Fatigue is a combination of reduced energy and a physical feeling of weariness. It may be predictable or come on unexpectedly and can interact with your sexual response in a variety of ways.

Many people believe that sex is supposed to be a super-duper workout each and every time. But unless you're bound for the Olympics sex does not have to be gymnastic, so you can take slowly the things we traditionally call romance, flirting, foreplay. Sex for us may not ever look like the beautiful people in the movies who are jumping each other's bones in fancy hotels, but our taking sex slow can be liberating, giving us the time to go easy and really feel what is happening.

This is great, of course, *if* we can find the energy to put these desires into play. Planning to have sex at a time when you are rested can be very helpful. Timing sex play to make sure you've got the energy to do what you want is also a good idea. Sometimes it takes creative thinking to fulfill your desires in ways that match your energy levels. Some wise people say that once you tap into your sexual energy you'll find energy you didn't know you had.

Mobility Considerations

Whether you're a quadriplegic and need assistance with positioning before you can have group sex, or someone with carpal tunnel syndrome who gets shooting pains when trying to masturbate, we all have different needs based on the kind of mobility we've got to work with. Many people think that a mobility restriction means no sex. We hope the ideas people with all sorts of mobility impairments share in this book will begin to dispel this myth, as it's one that not only the nondisabled buy into. Mobility restrictions mainly have an impact on the sexual behavior part of sexual response. They needn't have any impact whatsoever on arousal, desire, and fantasy. Fantasy can actually be used as a tool to problem solve mobility issues.

Communication Considerations

Not being able to communicate as "expected" means having to be a lot better at communicating than most people who don't live with a disability. Communication considerations include not only people who use augmentative communication, but also the vast range of language issues that can result from fatigue, medication, or cognitive disabilities. Having difficulties finding the right word, or trouble processing what we hear, can become a real challenge when it comes to sex play. Much "sex education" (a misnomer if ever there was one) comes from overhearing people talking about sex. If we can't hear what is said, or we can't put it into context, then we don't know as much about sex and sexual relationships as other people do. Written resources may be hard to understand, not available in Braille or on tape, or inaccessible to people who can't turn the pages, not to mention the fact that disability is seldom talked about in most basic materials. On the other hand, those of us who have had to maximize our nonverbal abilities can have an advantage with a partner. Many people find it hard to use words to communicate what they want sexually, and use their less developed nonverbal skills to try to tell their partners what they want.

Cognitive Considerations

Cognitive is just a fancy way of saying "thinking." Each of us has our own way of thinking. When something changes how we think, it can have an impact on our sexual fantasies, motivations, and feelings. Many things can interfere with your ability to think clearly, and everything that happens to you affects what you think about and often even *how* you think. Depression is one factor that can have a major impact on thinking. This illness can have devastating effects on a person's sexuality. It's essential to find ways of coping with cognitive issues that impede your connection to your sexuality. Cognitive issues can prevent you from even wanting to explore your sexuality. They can also be a problem during your exploration, as sexuality is such an intrinsic part of us that it invariably triggers things in us we weren't expecting.

Privacy

Environmental factors, particularly privacy, can also figure in sexual response. We find it difficult to allow ourselves to be relaxed and in a state where we can actually explore our sexual feelings when we know at any moment an unwanted person may intrude into our space. Other limits on privacy may influence our ability to create a space that's comfortable for exploration, or we may find limits on the kinds of explorations we can do unless we are given space of our own.

Sensation

Our ability to perceive stimuli is called *sensation*. It colors whether we feel a pinprick here or there, whether we're aware when our bladder is full, how much we can see or taste or hear. Sensation is involved with our sexual response in terms of what we can sense that turns us on. Sometimes we can "feel" something in a part of the body that lacks working nerve connections. This may be through fantasy or memory. Regardless of why we are feeling it, we think the feeling part is the most important. Every part of our bodies is represented somewhere in the brain. When an area that has no feeling has its brain part next to an area that does, sometimes stimulation of a feeling area can create a kind of sympathetic sensation in the unfeeling area as well.

Medications

> I started a new pill and within about two weeks I was feeling very unhappy about my work. I also wasn't thinking about sex at all. I didn't connect it to the medication. It seems silly, but because it was a tiny pill and I only took one a day it didn't even occur to me to think that it could be causing these things. But then I got changed to a different pill and within a couple of weeks I was back to my usual self, thinking about sex a lot, liking most parts of my job. So then I thought "Oh! That's what it was." I asked my doctor and he said, "That's a pretty rare side effect."

Most people who use medication as part of daily living know an awful lot about it: what type of drug it is, how much of it they take, what it feels like before and after taking it. But do you know about the effects

MEDICATION SIDE EFFECTS

Remember that no one experiences every side effect of a drug. Often, common side effects are experienced by about 20 percent of the people who take a medication, with varying degrees of severity. For some, side effects go away after a time.

Here are some common drug effects on sexuality:
- Decreased interest in sex (decreased libido): SSRIs and other antidepressants, timolol, spronolactone, propranalol, estrogen and progesterone, methyldopa, digoxin, doxipin, cisplain, cimetidine, chlorthalidone, chlorpormazine
- Difficulty having orgasms: SSRIs
- Decreased genital sensation: SSRIs
- Difficulty getting erections: SSRIs and other antidepressants, atenolol, baclofen, cimetidine, clonidine, digoxin, propranalol, spironolactone, other diuretics, timolol, hydralazine, haloperidol, naproxen, prazosin, progesterone, clofibrate, methadone, methyldopa
- Difficulty ejaculating: baclofen, SSRIs

Street drugs also have sexual side effects:
- Decreased interest in sex: speed, cocaine, diazepam, heroin, marijuana, PCP
- Difficulty getting erections: alcohol, speed, heroin, marijuana, nitrous oxide, PCP
- Difficulty having orgasms: speed, cocaine, heroin
- Difficulty ejaculating: speed, cocaine, diazepam, heroin, PCP

that meds have on your moods, thoughts, and sexuality? Probably not, unless you have figured it out by trial and error. Not much research has been done on this. When selective serotonin reuptake inhibitors (SSRIs, a type of depression medication) were first tested, the reported rate of sexual dysfunction was quite low. Now, though, this is known to be a fairly common side effect (felt in decreased libido, reduced sensation, painful orgasm, difficulty achieving orgasm, and so on). It isn't clear, however, that the investigators asked about sex, rather than just waiting for people to tell them about it. Drugs, both over-the-counter and street, can affect sex by increasing or decreasing blood flow, influencing the way we think, heightening or damping sensation or the perception of sensation, and elevating or lowering hormone levels (which can lead to changes in lubrication and libido). These effects can be either positive or negative. They can also be indirect. So someone on SSRIs may feel an improvement in libido as their depression lifts. Sexual pharmacology, or the ways that drugs interact with sexuality, is still a relatively new field. Chapter 14 lists some resources we can turn to for answers. If you can't get access to these books, you can direct your doctor to them so that you may find out if meds you're taking are affecting your sexuality, and if they are, whether alternatives are available. It may be difficult to talk to your doctor about this, especially if your doctor is in denial about your sexuality or does not think about this as an important aspect of your life. But it is often worth the effort.

Exercises

1. Make a list of things that are important to your sex life. This may (or may not) include other people, kissing, erections, lubrication, penetration, hugging, and feeling sexy. How has this changed over time? If you did not always live with your chronic illness or disability, would this list have been different before you acquired this disability? Do you think it will change in the future?

2. Throughout this chapter we have offered suggestions for small exercises designed to make you more aware of your sexual thoughts and feelings. This may be easier said than done. Many of us have been conditioned to ignore our sexuality, conditioned by parents, life experiences, religious figures, the media, or from living with pain that makes even finding a sexual thought a frustration. If you've been going through this chapter thinking none of this applies to you, you might start by looking at the ways you've been removed (or have removed yourself) from communicating with yourself sexually.

3. Write a short story of your life and your sexual response. It doesn't have to be fancy or on paper; you can do it in your head. Think about the earliest time you can remember feeling sexy and the messages you got about it. What are the messages you got from doctors, parents, teachers, peers, about being attractive, attracted to others, sexual in any way? If you've had to deal with the medical establishment your whole life, chances are pretty fair that you've experienced some form of abuse related to your body (from an inappropriate comment to being assaulted, and anything in between). What are the messages you took from those experiences?

Communication

You may have looked at the title of this chapter and thought, "Communication? I want a chapter about *sex!*" Hold on there. This chapter is actually very practical, and definitely about sex. It is almost impossible to have good sex without good communication. A lot of good sex is in fact nothing more than good communication, cybersex being only the most recent example of this. Any sex expert will tell you that the biggest sex organ is the brain, and even though this sounds like a cliché it's true.

What's to be gained by becoming better sex communicators? In addition to improving our chances of getting what we want, we also get closer to our partners. Because it can be so hard to communicate about sex, if we get good at it we are likely to improve our general communication skills as well. In addition to all this, sexual communication can be seen as a political act. If we look like we live with a disability, we aren't supposed to be having sex…and we certainly shouldn't be so bold as to talk about it. By pushing the boundaries of this stereotype we force people to confront their bigoted (or merely ignorant) notions about anyone who looks like they live with a disability. We may even challenge our own notions of disability and what living with one or with a chronic illness means.

> *I gave up on talking to my family about it when I was a kid, but I'll still sometimes make a comment, or just start talking about sex with certain people because I know it gets a rise out of them. They just never expect it from me because of the way I look. I like the fact that it pisses people off a little and makes them squirm.*

Communication requires several steps. The first is knowing what it is you want to communicate, which means understanding what you want or need sexually. This step is really about talking with yourself, carrying on a dialogue that brings you to a clearer picture of what you want. The exercises at the end of chapter 3 contained a suggestion that you make a list of things that are important to your sex life. That list is a good place to start. Sexual fantasy can be a rich element in this process. If you can, give yourself permission to fantasize about any sexual possibility, knowing that many ideas will come and go through your head, and that many people enjoy fantasizing about doing things that they wouldn't actually want to do. To be able to tell someone what we need and want out of a sexual experience, we ought to have some idea of what we need and want, to begin with. We don't want to make this sound easy. Everyone has a hard time communicating their sexual needs. We haven't even found that it gets a whole lot easier the more we do it. The only thing we can say for sure is that without telling someone what you want sexually you are *very* unlikely to get it from them by chance. It'd be like expecting to win the lottery without picking a set of numbers and buying a ticket.

The next step is figuring out how you are going to get this message across. At this point, most sex guides say something like, "So what you have to do is sit down with your partner, talk with them, express your feelings, desires, inhibitions," and so on. But, of course, we don't all sit down and talk easily. Communication happens in a dozen different ways, and what we need to do is find out how we communicate best; how we feel most confident, comfortable, and safe; and then use that method as much as possible.

> As an AAC user, there is one thing that has always frustrated me in developing a personal and intimate relationship, or even a simple friendship. Having to use a voice output system device, or a display letter board, often does not reveal my true self or my true identity. My personality and character traits are muffled by a monotone voice or a display that is slow and tedious in responding. This leaves me with little free-flowing dialogue and social interaction. Also, what most people seem to forget is the sound of a person's own voice does attract people. Without an authentic-sounding voice, it is hard to attract people from the opposite sex. I think this specific issue is often overlooked by speech therapists, although there is still the lack of technology that may solve this problem. However, it does need to be raised, and talked about.

Most of us tend to overvalue talking and undervalue all other ways of communicating. Facial expressions, screaming, moaning, moving, gazing, whistling, blowing, laughing, and crying are all ways of saying things. Even if spoken language is not possible, it's still important and possible to communicate in many ways.

Now put your plan into action, letting a potential partner know what you want them to know. An important part of this is making sure the person you want to talk to is paying attention *and* that the way you communicate can work for them as well as you. At first you might need to check in with them about how they are understanding what you're saying, how they are feeling about it, and so forth. This process goes back and forth, getting clearer (you hope) at each stage. It is always helpful to summarize things at the end, with words, gestures, or looks, to make sure that everyone understood the conversation in the same way. We consider good communication to be consensual—meaning all the people involved in the conversation have agreed to have it and they all try to make sure everyone can equally understand what's being said.

The last stage is, of course, being willing to hear a response. Communication, as we'll say again and again, is a two-way street (or it could be a three- or four-way street, depending on how many people you're involved with!). Getting up the energy and often courage to say something is one thing, but being willing to hear a response that may not be the one we want to hear is another thing entirely.

Barriers to Good Sexual Communication

So there I was, about to have my very first sexual experience with another person, and he says to me, "Tell me exactly what you want." I didn't have a clue what I wanted, I just knew that I was aching for something. And even if I had had a clearer idea, I don't think I could have said anything, I would have been too embarrassed.

In our survey, many people told us they would hesitate to initiate a conversation for fear of confusing a partner, hurting a partner's feelings, or being anxious that they already ask for too much from a partner and don't feel "right" adding to that burden. In addition, some may hesitate to communicate what they want or need sexually because of problems in their relationship.

Myths

The idea that sex should be spontaneous and that talking about it will make it "clinical" or spoil the mood is a major barrier to communicating about sex. We've already discussed the myth that sex is something that comes naturally and doesn't need to be talked about with a partner. This is a very powerful, but confusing, myth in our culture. We are surrounded everywhere by information that is supposed to make us better sex partners. Listen to talk radio, watch TV talk shows and infomercials, read the newspaper or magazines—someone is always ready to tell us how to do sex better. It's almost expected these days that we should want to improve ourselves as lovers. But talking honestly and openly with the people we're going to have sex with is still rarely mentioned. We're supposed to learn how to do it ahead of time and surprise our partner. There is the implicit idea that to be a good lover we must somehow know what a partner wants before they have a chance to ask, and we shouldn't have to talk about what turns us on because your partner should know. There is little support for us to really talk about sex or sexuality, to speak honestly about our desires.

Negative Beliefs

Our own and others' beliefs and biases about sexuality can get in the way of communication. Growing up, we have all received messages about sex. If you were raised believing that you had no right to your own sexual desires, no right to your own body even, that your body was the property of doctors who were busy fixing you and that your desires were something you needed to get rid of, or were a luxury, all these factors can make it difficult for you to share sexual thoughts with others or even yourself. Most of us think that other people have an easier time talking about sexuality. But with a few exceptions, we're all raised with some sex-negative beliefs. So when any two of us get together the results can range from unbearable to embarrassing to comical to great.

Extra expectations can be placed on anyone living with a disability. When we don't look like everyone else, or if we can't keep up with the speed of a conversation in a fast restaurant, or we can't go to a specific dance club because it's too smoky, nondisabled people tend to have an expectation that we will educate others about our differences. Sometimes this happens in a nice "gee, that's fascinating, tell me more" way, sometimes in an annoyed "why can't you be like everyone else?" way. Either way, one underlying message is that we are too much trouble, and it shouldn't be others' responsibility to make change. The message is that we're different and thus it's our responsibility to communicate all they need to know. Rarely do nondisabled people take the responsibility for their biases.

Sexual Information and Vocabulary

Many of us lack basic information about our bodies, desires, and sexual response. Sometimes we don't even have the language to discuss it. It's a bit like trying to talk about mathematics but not knowing any numbers. The situation is even worse than this, because we don't just have a lack of information, we have *mis*information. Much of what we learn from the mainstream media is inaccurate or misleading. If all we know about sex is what we learned on television, then communicating with someone about our sexuality becomes very difficult. Some of us did not have access to the same kinds of sex education our peers did (and the sex education *they* received was hardly adequate). Very few of us are raised knowing the actual words for all our body parts, or being able to discuss them without shame or guilt.

One of us works in a sex toy store and sees this all the time with nondisabled people as much as with people living with disabilities. People come into the store, obviously interested in buying a sex toy, and clearly wanting help, but they don't know how to ask. Some of this comes from embarrassment but often it's because they simply don't know what to ask for (since most of us don't know the finer details of sex toy lingo). Because they don't have a sex toy vocabulary, people end up flustered and will often leave without talking at all unless they are approached by someone friendly who can offer them the words to ask their questions. A lot of people who use augmentative or alternative communication may simply not have the symbols or the words to communicate about sex at all. Even when they have a keyboard to spell words out, they still need to know the words first.

Privacy

Another barrier to communicating about sex is privacy. Most of us have been taught that sexuality is a private matter. This can be another trap, because it leads to the idea that if you don't have privacy you can't have sex. Later on in this chapter we offer some tips on communicating about sex with little or no privacy. Privacy is hard to find, particularly for people who are living with their parents, in a group home, or in other institutional settings. But there are some private places we can have for our-selves, the most obvious being our mind.

> *I remember clearly the moment (I was sixteen years old) when I finally realized that I had a whole fantasy life that was completely unrelated to my outside life, that it was a good thing, a sign that I had a healthy and active mind. I live in many worlds, some of them with complete story lines, and I can do all kinds of things in my fantasy worlds. For a while I think I worried that my parents could read my mind, but knowing that no one can do that gives me a huge amount of freedom.*

Often we're told that an active fantasy life is something to be ashamed of. It's childish, we're told, and fantasy is only for people who are afraid to experience reality. But fantasy is *not* childish, and our fan-tasy life is a wonderful, private world. It will be the only private space that some people ever get. If you have a partner, it is up to you to decide whether to invite them in, and into which parts of you and your fantasy world. Making time for yourself, then, and clearing your head of other things to make time to think about sex, can be an important tactic in dealing with a lack of privacy.

Blaming the Disability

Having something to blame for your communications problems can become a barrier because then you don't have to work to change them. When nondisabled people get into a relationship and quickly find they don't know how to communicate about sex, they don't really know where to turn for someone to blame. Often they say they work too much, maybe one of them has a drug problem, maybe it's the kids, or the mortgage, or maybe it's just that they are from two different planets (which is the stupidest pop psychology of them all). The blame never gets put where it should, squarely between the two of them and their inability to communicate with each other. And because it's all about blame and not about solutions, often they don't even realize that communication is something you can learn to do better. It's not about our "nature." It's about learning how to communicate (which means both giving *and* receiving information). In a relationship where one or both people has a disability, there's the perfect scapegoat. Just as disability is often considered the cause of all our other personality characteristics ("she's such a brave quad!," "he's such a jerk, but I guess I'd be the same way if I was blind"), it can quickly become the excuse for things going poorly in a relationship. To have healthy communication, it is crucial to be aware of when the disability is being used as an excuse not to communicate or as justification for poor communication. Whether the relationship has one or two people who identify as disabled, usually both people use the disability excuse at one time or another. This can be very tricky because it is unlikely that a sensitive nondisabled partner will call you on using your disability as an excuse, as they will probably feel like they have no right. We all make excuses sometimes, and we need to try not to hide behind the disability, even though we may have learned that this can be a useful survival tool. Disabilities can sometimes result in communication problems merely because of their own dynamics. Fatigue and pain in particular can make a sustained communication effort difficult. Being in a relationship with someone who hasn't yet learned to easily understand how you speak also poses some challenges.

Confusing Needs, Desires, and Requirements

Sometimes we need to separate communication about the sexual aspects of relationships from other kinds of communication, or these discussions can get lost among other relationship stuff. We all tend to shy away from talking about sex, and a preoccupation with other aspects of a relationship can help us avoid the topic. This isn't great for any sexual relationship, but it really doesn't work if communication is a requirement of having sex. If we need to tell a partner about positions, or if we require assistance undressing, we must communicate. Not doing so means not having sex with others at all, having unsafe sex with other people, or having lousy sex with someone.

When I'm having a date with my partner and my attendant isn't here it's always like, "I need this, I need that." Sometimes I feel really demanding, so then maybe I'm kind of shy about saying, "I need you to touch me, I need to touch you."

One way we often let our sexuality get muddled with other aspects of our lives is when we confuse daily needs with sexual needs and desires. Many people who are in relationships, and whose partners help them with some aspect of care, talk about how difficult it is to be sexual with someone who just tied your shoe laces, or wiped food off your face. Why is it supposed to be sexy to watch a Hollywood movie where a woman is wiping cream off a man's face and yet it's the opposite of sexy when our partner removes crumbs from our beard because we can't? Is it about power? Freedom? Control? Maybe it's only sexy when unrealistically good-looking people do it. Maybe it's about our inability to be in more than one role at one time ("don't try to flirt with me now, because right now I'm 'taking care of your needs' ").

When some needs are considered more important than others, a hierarchy can be created in a relationship. There may be an unspoken rule that it's not okay to flirt with your partner while they are doing the dishes or making the bed. The need for both partners to flirt, to be playful, becomes secondary to the daily living stuff. It can also happen that help with dressing, answering the phone, running for a cab, or cooking become the only way one partner can meet the other's needs. We may think that, because we need to ask a partner for help getting dressed, we shouldn't ask them to be more open about what turns them on. Letting our partners off the hook from the responsibility to create an honest sexual relationship because they help with dressing or other things has a negative impact on the relationship. Note the difference between your asking for help with something and wanting to engage in a two-way conversation about what's happening between yourself and your partner.

I know that there have been times when I've been in a relationship with nondisabled lovers and I've not always been able to talk to them openly about how I'm feeling because they're providing some kind of support outside of the sexual relationship. It feels like that relationship gets put into different compartments depending on what is happening at that time. I feel at times that I might be burdening them with having them attend to one more thing. It doesn't feel good when I get into that space because then we both lose out on having an honest discussion, and also I might be feeling horny and then the moment is lost because they're doing something else for me.

In any relationship there is interdependence. The balance can shift from day to day, but there are always things that each person gets, or needs to get from the other. Too often, in a relationship between someone living with a disability and a nondisabled partner, the disabled person is perceived as being dependent on the other, yet the ways in which the nondisabled person is dependent are seldom acknowledged. Our needs can come to be seen as overwhelming while our partners' demands are hidden or viewed as minimal, or are even addressed elsewhere, outside the relationship.

Creating Positive Communication

Good communication has to start with you. We've said this before and we're saying it again because it's so important. In most sex manuals, communication is written about as if it is something that we can isolate from the relationship as a whole. But it is impossible to examine the issue of communicating with a lover without looking at the relationship in general. Working on your sexuality—exploring, asking questions, moving forward—invariably means working on other aspects of your life.

Communicating with a potential or current partner about sex has taken a lot of practice, and I think is difficult for TABs as well! As a young woman I was so embarrassed about my artificial leg that I couldn't talk about it at all—just hoped they'd already noticed or something and used to dread the moment I would take it off— urrgghhh...I still cringe, remembering. But these days I've become very forthright and have come to the conclusion that if my prospective lover can't handle HEARING about what works for me, then they won't handle DOING it either. Of course I like to work up to this, not blurt it all out on first meeting a potential partner, but definitely while fooling around with each other's bodies, I like to talk about both my body's peculiarities, and the things my body enjoys. Boldness is best.

Many of the people who filled out our survey told us that living with a disability has enhanced their sexual communication. Disability can allow us the opportunity for creativity and the chance to see ourselves as being different from the impossible role model. In this way disability can become a catalyst for a kind of change and growth that nondisabled people usually can't imagine.

It has made me creative and adaptable. Many nondisabled people have very boring sex lives. Mine is a long ways from boring. Also, communications in general are better because of having to communicate about my disability.

I guess that [communication] has enhanced [my sex life] because I pay attention to what feels good for me and my partner. I have learned several secrets to pleasing a man by asking questions and reacting to the answers.

They say sex is a lot about communication. If this is true, my disability does force me to talk to my partners much more than I would, left to my own devices. I have to talk about what we're going to do, what needs to happen in order to do it, what I can and can't do. So there's little possibility of anonymous sex.

Boundaries

By boundaries we mean defining where you begin and end. What your needs, desires, and fears are...and what they aren't. If someone who makes jokes when they feel nervous isn't aware that they do this, they might find themselves in a situation where a friend feels they were being made fun of. The unaware person may see their friend as too sensitive, or as misinterpreting a comment. The person who is aware that they do this will realize that their nervousness contributed to this situation, and be able to take some responsibility. This may seem like an obvious example, but it's important to remember that this happens with disability issues all the time.

One benefit to knowing your own boundaries is that it can help you notice when other people's issues are being foisted onto you. Take the following example:

Jack and Richard have been dating for about four months. Their relationship was sexual from the beginning. Richard lives with chronic back pain that usually takes him out of commission one or two days a week. Jack is nondisabled, and has been complaining lately that Richard isn't as affectionate as he used to be, and Jack is questioning Richard's interest.

It may sound as though Jack is unsympathetic to Richard's pain. He can't understand the way chronic pain can affect almost every aspect of life. Maybe, Jack thinks, Richard's pain is getting worse because he is unhappy with the relationship. Or maybe it isn't his pain at all, but Richard is really just pulling away from Jack.

Another interpretation is that Jack is understanding. That he doesn't expect Richard to be able to jump up and hug him every time he walks through the door. But that after repeated attempts to get Richard to talk about his feelings about the relationship, or about his chronic pain, Jack is now getting tired of trying. Maybe Richard isn't communicating at all with Jack.

Because we don't have more information, we could interpret this scenario many ways. But when there is poor communication, the people in the relationship also don't have all the information they need. Whenever we have to fill in the blanks of how the other person feels, we're in trouble because we usually fill in those blanks with our own issues. One of the great benefits of clarifying our boundaries and knowing what we want is that we can clearly understand at least half the story. A result of good boundaries is that you can begin to share the responsibility for good communication. Communication goes in both directions and should not be the responsibility of just one person.

When Do I Talk About My Disability?

> I had decided that the sexual side of my life was over and had resigned myself to that. Now, at sixty-four, I am in love for the first time. I met the man on the Internet in a "chatroom" three years ago.... Before him, I'd indulged in cyber affairs with a number of men. At first I did not tell them I was disabled as I didn't plan to ever meet them. That got too complicated. Finally I came out of the closet. This is before I had actually met my future love in person. I sent an email to my chat friends, telling them. The email response from my future lover was "... and your point is...?" I almost fell in love with him right then.

There are at least two issues to think about related to the question of talking about disability. First, what do you want to say about your disability, and second, when do you want to say it. People living with disabilities are invariably put in the position of being "The Ambassadors of Disability." Because nondisabled people have so many hang-ups about disability, and so little information, if we choose to have sex with nondisabled people we do much of the initiating of conversations. That doesn't mean that we should disclose more information than we feel comfortable with. We aren't required to tell our entire medical history or the story of our life to someone we are going to be sexual with. The information we give should be based on what we both want and need them to know so that we can have good and safe sex with them.

There's also the question of timing disability information. When to tell? As is our constant refrain, there is no right answer here. The decision is yours. Consider some of the following situations.

Nick was in a car accident two years ago. His pelvis was broken badly and he had injuries to his bladder. He now catheterizes regularly. Tanya met Nick at a party and asked him out on a date. They've gone out a couple of times and she has been flirting with him. She goes over to his apartment to watch a movie and asks if she can spend the night. Nick hasn't told her anything about his disability.

Pedro has been blind since birth. He split up with his girlfriend last year and is now looking for a new relationship. He hasn't met anyone he is really interested in through friends or activities, so he is thinking of placing an ad in the personals section of the paper. He isn't sure if he should mention his disability.

Cynthia has cerebral palsy and uses a Bliss board to communicate. She lives in a group home. She really likes Brad (who also lives in the home). When they get a chance, they make out, but they are not supposed to and the workers rarely leave them alone. She has masturbated before on her own and she likes clitoral stimulation. She has tried vaginal penetration but it hurt. She wants to tell Brad that she wants to have sex with him, but not intercourse. But she doesn't have the Bliss vocabulary she needs to tell him this, and doesn't know how to spell it all. Also, she is worried about what Brad will think about this—maybe he won't want to have sex with her without intercourse.

Michele has had cybersex with a number of people, writing hot emails back and forth and in chatrooms. She has maintained a correspondence with one person who now wants to meet her in person. She likes her, but thinks maybe she won't meet her because she doesn't know how to tell her that she has a colostomy.

There are no absolute rules for disclosure. Rob Kocur, a quad for the past eighteen years, wrote an article in *New Mobility* about personal ads. He conducted an experiment, placing two ads in his local paper. In the first ad he did not disclose his disability and in the second ad he did. He got more responses to the first ad. At first he suggests that people living with disabilities not disclose because it would drastically decrease the number of responses. Leaving the disability out at least gives you the chance on the phone of being a person first, letting them communicate with you without all their baggage about disability. But some people are fiercely proud of their disability and don't want to hide it. For others the rejection after rapport has been established is more disappointing than an initial rejection because of the word *disability* in the ad. As Kocur concludes, "why not see the disability as a tool for weeding out those people who don't really belong in your life, anyway?"

Sometimes being upfront about my disability can mean taking a risk, and it's disappointing when that person makes a decision not to maintain contact, but I'd rather not have to always second-guess if someone is going to be able to handle it, and I'd rather know right away.

I hear other women speak of sexual objectification by men, but that's not usually something I encounter. Most men seem to see me as asexual or "one of the guys." That was harder for me to deal with when I was single and in the "dating market." Of course, if a guy couldn't see me as a full human being, sexuality and all, I knew he was a jerk that wasn't worth my time."

We have to consider our emotional state when deciding when to disclose. You don't want to let someone know about your disability on a day when your cat's in the hospital, the government is harassing you, and your favorite plant just died. You may also want to consider how the other person is going to take the information in. While it's not our responsibility to cater to nondisabled people's phobias about disability, it's good to remember that it takes everyone time to adjust to any kind of difference. People with an acquired disability already know this and may be able to relate a little. It may be harder to imagine for people who have always lived with their disability. Considering this may simply mean disclosing in a way that makes a potential partner feel they can take some time without appearing to be the cruel monster. If a relationship is going to work, everyone involved has to be able to communicate without fear of being judged quickly. There is a big difference between someone saying, "I'm afraid of what it means that you're disabled" and someone saying, "I can't imagine ever being in relationship or having sex with someone who is disabled." The latter comment is so often expressed, and the first so seldom, that it's easy to confuse the two.

Trying not to make assumptions about other people's knowledge or comfort levels is hard, but vital to establishing a relationship. Disability adds an extra dimension, making negotiations almost like being in a cross-cultural relationship. It's not that we and the person we're with are so fundamentally different. We both have feelings, experiences, thoughts, and fears. It's the individual experiences that are different, and the ways we communicate about them.

Although the responsibility is shared, we shouldn't take a balance sheet approach to relationships. It doesn't help if one person starts adding up all the things they do. Maybe he (or she) does most of the cooking, or most of the financial dealings, and then when it is time to talk about sex, he may take the attitude that he does *all* these other things, so it's not fair to expect him, at the end of his long day, to actively engage in a conversation about sex. This may be just a way of avoiding talking about sex, or it may be an expression of resentment that they have to do so much.

> *I keep feeling that I probably shouldn't be asking for the help I want, that I should really be doing it myself, and that maybe I don't deserve a pain crisis where I can't get from my bed to the bathroom, but other people don't deserve to have me as their responsibility. I get caught up in self-recrimination. I blame myself for not doing enough, but find myself with no reliable idea of what I can really do. And the consequences of overdoing can be so disastrous, that I just can't push myself the way I normally do. The fear really is paralyzing.*

In a sexual relationship where one partner needs more assistance than the other, and that other partner takes responsibility for providing assistance, it can become an excuse to avoid a conversation they simply don't want to have. "I'm not going to talk about being cold to you in bed, I have to go do the laundry." "I don't want to talk about oral sex, I need to get you undressed and help you into bed."

Relationships aren't balance sheets. Doing the dishes and talking about our sexual fantasies aren't linked (unless you have sexual fantasies about doing the dishes!). A sexual relationship won't work well if people aren't willing to talk to each other. What is usually happening in these situations is that one partner doesn't want to talk about sex because of their discomfort with the topic, but they use the disability as an excuse.

Everyone involved needs to be vigilant about this. If one person is really doing too much assistance, then work on that problem. Can you get a PCA? Can you schedule a sex talk for when no one needs to help anyone with anything?

Timing

It's a good idea to plan some private time just to talk about sex. Ideally, we talk about sex before starting a sexual relationship. Talking about safer sex, birth control, and whatever other information (positioning, bowel and bladder routines) you think you need to share is not always a sexy experience. True, it can be informative and fun, but having it during a moment of intimacy can be distracting and a turn-off.

> I remember once insisting on having the "sex talk" right before we were going to have sex. I wanted to talk about condoms and find out if she used another kind of birth control. The conversation took an unexpected turn and she told me if she ever got pregnant by accident she would have the baby. I was only twenty-two at the time and there was no way I was ready to be a father. After the conversation we started fooling around, and even though I thought she was totally hot, and the rest of me was very turned on, I couldn't get an erection at all. I think my body had heard what she said and got very scared off. After that I learned to time the "sex talk" a little differently!

Take Initiative and Practice

Seizing the initiative and making your interest known is very hard, but somebody's got to do it. Because none of us feel that comfortable talking about sex, we get quite good at avoiding it. A nondisabled person may live a *lifetime* without talking about sex honestly. So if we want to get some, we may have to start the conversation. Consider practicing. Practice with a friend, practice with yourself in front of a mirror. If you're going to communicate verbally it's good to choose what words you're most comfortable with and practice getting the words out. If you're going to do it nonverbally, practice whichever way you communicate. Type out an email ahead of time and go through it. Figure out what you want to say in your head first and then be creative about how to communicate it in a conversation. This book can be an ideal conversation starter. Simply by having it around (since you've already got a copy, we can say this without its seeming like a marketing scheme!) you are letting people around you know that you are interested in sex, interested in thinking and talking about it, and you may be interested in having it (we don't want to be presumptuous).

Flirting

What I worked out is that attraction and flirtation is the greatest game of tease and bluff and that anyone with a good sense of humor, dressed attractively, and out for fun will get their hands— or in my case hand—on just about anyone they want. The perfect body is only important to shallow twats that no one but other shallow twats want anyway. I don't know whether I ever would have worked this out if it hadn't been for my best buddies in my youth theater days.

I love to flirt. It gives me this feeling of being noticed and makes me feel energized. I flirt with lots of people of both sexes (I'm not bisexual). It is a great way to pass time and sometimes it does lead to something interesting. I can flirt without getting involved, but I can't get involved without flirting.

What Is Flirting?

You're flirting when you make a playfully romantic or sexual overture to someone you're interested in. There are a couple of key points in this definition. First: Flirting is supposed to be playful—it shouldn't be torture. While it may take some time to warm up to how much fun it can be for you, keep this in mind: Sooner than you think, you'll be having a ball regardless of whether the person you're interested in feels the same way. Second: Flirting can be about romance, sex, or just fun, depending on what your goals are: All you have to do is learn how to communicate these goals clearly with others. Once you get going in the wonderful world of flirting, you'll find your own truth within it. We asked a few expert flirters to share some tips with us.

Be You

Don't try to be someone you're not—after all, if you try to be someone else to get a date, sooner or later the other person will figure it out. Instead, focus on being proud and pleased with the kind of person you are now, and communicating that to those around you. Most of all, make sure you're in a good mood when you're getting ready to go out flirting. The best flirts have a strong sense of fun and are playful, adventurous, and incredibly curious about those around them.

Be Bold

Don't be afraid to make the first move! You'd be amazed at how relieved most folks are to have someone else do it—remember, you're not the only one who's shy. Try practicing on folks you're not romantically or sex- ually interested in but whom you encounter on a daily basis, just to get used to making small talk with strangers. Next time you're in line at the bank, say, "Nice tie" or "I really love your haircut" to the person ahead of you. Most of all, be sincere—people can spot insincerity a mile away. Remember that flirting is a skill like any other, so it takes a while to get good at it—and different things work with different people.

Be Involved

Feel as though you don't know anybody to flirt with? That you only see the same people all the time, and you already know you aren't interested in dating them? You can flirt with anyone; it's good practice. So get out there and get busy meeting new folks. Think about what you enjoy doing and try doing it in a more social setting. For example, if you like painting, take some art classes at your local community center, or if you like team sports join a local recreational team. Remember, the more people you meet (and therefore flirt with) the more likely you are to meet one whom you'll want to take home with you.

Be Noticeable

Many of us have spent a lot of our lives trying or even expecting *not* to be noticed by those around us. Well, when you're on a flirt hunt it's time to get out the flirting props! Put some jazzy bumper stickers on your chair, wear a slogan T-shirt or something that invites those around you to comment on it or engage you in conversation. After all, shy folks need a reason to talk to you—might as well give them one.

Be Clear

Flirting can be just nonserious practice flirting, or it can be headed down romantic or sexual avenues. That means you need to be clear before you head into possible flirting situations about what you do—and don't—want. Looking for a fun, ego-building exchange with someone else? Looking for sex? A date? A new friend? What your goals are will affect the signals you send, as well as the responses you get.

Be Approachable

While it's not a bad idea to go out with friends you feel comfortable with on a flirt hunt, since you're a lot more likely to be your own vivacious best self, it's also important that you not be constantly in their company. If your friends surround you all the time it's a lot harder for someone to approach you. Make sure you have time both with and away from your group of friends, so you can spend more time looking at those around you for lovely prospects and also so that anyone who's been checking you out has a better chance of getting next to you.

Be Polite

Given that rejection is a normal part of any flirting process, it's important to treat those who approach us the way we'd like to be treated if we were to take the risk of being first to break the ice. After all, interest is a compliment, and deserves to be treated as such. A polite but clear "Thank you, that's very sweet of you, but no" is more than appropriate in any situation.

Be Interested

Once you've established contact with someone, it's always good practice to focus on asking them open-ended questions about themselves. It gives you a chance to hear a bit about how they think about things and what they like to do with their time—all important information for you in terms of deciding just how interested you are. And whatever you do, don't fall into the common trap of ignoring the people you're interested in out of your worry that you'll find out they aren't interested in you. Remember that rejection is all part of the process, and it's not necessarily personal. So if you see someone who looks interesting to you, don't be so afraid of rejection that you never take a chance—smile at them! After all, you're not declaring your undying love, you're just letting them see you've noticed them and are pleased with what you see.

Be Sensitive

Some folks are space invaders, so that even when they don't know you that well they are much more physically close, or in your space, than is comfortable for you. Others seem really distant, and even cold, no matter how well they know you. Each individual person has a different sense of personal space, or amount of physical room they want in an exchange with someone else. It's also true that the amount of space folks prefer is affected by culture and practice, as are other means of physical signaling like eye contact or touching the person you are with while talking. Try to take your cue from the person you're with—learning to be sensitive to their boundaries will go a long way toward their wanting to keep talking to you and greatly increases the odds you'll get somewhere with them.

Be Honest

Don't agree to give someone your phone number out of pity, or not wanting to hurt their feelings. If you're polite about your refusals, you've done as much as you need to, no matter how pulled you are to "take care" of them. While you may feel mean doing it, it's actually more likely to hurt them if you pretend to be interested when you're not, as their hopes would actually get even higher that the two of you might end up dating. After all, wouldn't you rather know right away if someone isn't interested? That way you can get on with flirting with someone who is.

Communicating Without Privacy

We all do quite a bit of our communicating in public, but when it comes to talking about sex, most people need privacy. This can be a hard thing to find when living in any kind of institutional setting. Even if there aren't actual rules against privacy, there are usually many unspoken restrictions on having time alone or having time with one other person. Even non-verbal communication can be intercepted easily.

When two people have infrequent privacy, they can use some of this time together to develop a code, so that in more public encounters they can arrange meetings, say what they would like to do, or express feelings. This is pretty limited, as you have to be able to remember all the codes. When using words or signs, try linking them to familiar things. The name of something you hate can be the code for feeling angry, the name of a sexy star or a TV show could mean you are thinking about having sex.

If you can write, then passing notes is another option, although you have to be careful to dispose of them so they won't be read by other people. People are less likely to go through bathroom garbage than other garbage, so throwing out ripped-up notes in the bathroom is one possibility.

Communicating About Pain

I try to let my partner know what I like. It is hard because sometimes I can handle something, and other times that same thing is impossible for me to handle.

Pain, whether you have it all the time or it comes and goes, can be devastating to your sexuality. It is difficult to try to explain major pain, the sense of urgency it causes, and its aftereffects to someone who has never felt it.

There is often a spoken or unspoken belief that everyone gets what they deserve and that pain is something that is deserved, imagined, or not all that bad. When people who don't have pain believe this, then they feel protected, knowing that it can't happen to them. So they won't be very open to understanding pain.

Rather than trying to explain the pain well enough so that the other person will understand it (this is close to impossible), it is often better to talk about the effects it has. Pain may interfere with our feeling we're a sexual person, as it may make us feel not "at home" in our bodies, make it hard for us to feel sexy, make it difficult for us to reach out physically or emotionally, and sap our energy. Pain may be predictable, with times of the day that are better than others, or things that can lead to temporary relief. Sex itself can also cause pain, or make it worse.

It has to be clear to both partners that the person experiencing the pain or limitation because of a disability is the one who knows best. We must say when something hurts, and if we don't then things are fine. This is a big commitment from both sides: to be honest about what we are feeling, and to believe the messages we are getting. Guilt about causing pain should be discussed.

You need to expect the unexpected. What sends us into fits of ecstasy one week can cause extreme pain the next. Communicating "in the moment" is essential. If verbal communication is difficult, then clear signals are crucial. Here we're borrowing from the world of S/M with its "safewords." Establishing signals for *yes, no, more, less,* and *stop* can make communicating during sex play much easier. Use of signals can be useful even for people who are verbal. For more aspects of S/M play that relate to dealing with pain see chapter 11.

Meeting People

At twenty-six I have discovered that dancing on my knees and flirting with other men is fun. I get into most gay bars by getting other men to assist me up the stairs with my chair when possible. Or if I go to a nightclub I just stay in one spot upstairs dancing on my knees. My favorite line is, "I am faking this disability for the view." I am a gay male and I find that accessibility is an issue for going to dance clubs and bars. In the past I had found that in some dance clubs I was kicked off the dance floor for taking up too much space. Or I was told it is too dangerous for me to dance on my knees. I was even called a horny geriatric in the local gay newspaper. I believe the exact words were: "What I want to know is who is the horny geriatric who conveniently parks his able walker in front of the club." I was twenty-three at the time. I informed the newspaper that I was definitely not a horny geriatric. Even if I was, what would be wrong with that? It is getting better as I keep on getting out.

Friends, family, and partners have all been supportive, but most care services are still designed to function as if the disabled are "invalid" or "shut-in." For example, wheelchair repair services are notoriously slow and ineffectual and—even in urban areas—there are limited transportation services. I must often limit my socializing at clubs, or even private parties, to avoid being stranded by missing the last bus.

Work in the media! No, seriously, you have to be out there, in the real world, meeting a lot of people, getting used to being stared at and staring 'em down. My disabled friends who spend all their time going to and from small workplaces and not getting out and about, get very little action. It really helps to feel confident and bold.

A FEW TIPS ON CHOOSING PARTNERS

Some people are attracted to potential partners because they seem danger-ous. The risk-taking element can be exciting at first. But in the long run, dangerous partners can be dangerous both mentally and physically.

While there are absolutely no foolproof ways to choose a partner, here are some things to consider:

- What is their track record? Ask about previous relationships, how they are described, how they ended. You can also find out a lot by how a person's friends describe them.

- While you can't judge a person by their family, asking about family can sometimes give you a glimpse into the way they were raised, and how they might do it differently (if you're looking for a potential long-term part-ner this could be important).

- Ask yourself, would you trust this person in other ways? Would you buy a used car from them? Do their friends seem to trust them?

- Are they looking for the same things you are? If you're seeking a fast and clean relationship based solely on hot sex, but they're scoping out baby strollers and table settings, you may want to back off.

- What are their boundaries like? Usually if someone professes their undy-ing love for you at the end of a first date, well, there may be issues worth looking into there.

Over and over in response to our survey people wrote about the main prob-lem's being not how to have sex, but whom to have sex with. Lack of avail-able partners, not a lack of creative solutions for what to do with those partners, is the main issue for many people. Where to meet people is a huge obstacle, and any suggestions may seem like pat answers. Standard advice (smile, be more friendly, look more outgoing, try to make an effort) does not acknowledge that many people are afraid to get involved with a disabled person. Sometimes the ideas and suggestions may be useful, but when they are couched in terms of our inadequacy they defeat the purpose.

Some of us spent our younger years avoiding other people living with disabilities, not wanting to be typecast, feeling that if we had a disabled friend then people would think we only want disabled friends. We may have missed out on opportunities for some great friendships.

When we get involved with someone else with a disability, there can be both advantages and pitfalls. They may already "speak the same language," that is, understand about disability issues, not need to be educated about things. On the other hand, we can't assume that they know anything about our disability. We have to be careful not to get into competition about who is the most disabled. But the chances are higher that their living space will be accessible. There may be some similarities of experiences or issues that won't come from having a nondisabled lover.

Most of the lovers I have had are people who have disabilities. It has been my experience that because both of us are coming to the relationship from a more equal ground, that there are fewer power imbalances that play themselves out. We both know what is possible sexually and what isn't and, where possible, talk together openly about how to make it work for both of us. One lover was a man who was very open to talking to me about my concerns and fears. Many of my fears were about what I was able to do to satisfy him as well as other things that were related to my disability which might have "turned off" other lovers, such as maybe having an accident in bed or seeing a body that wasn't like Demi Moore. He was very sensitive and caring about how I felt and also was able to relate to his own earlier sexual experiences and feeling uncertain. Our sexual relationship was wonderful for the time it lasted and was very creative in ways that I wonder would be possible with a nondisabled lover who didn't have firsthand experience with disability.

I have a lot of disabilities—that means that I depend on attendant services for a great deal of my care. When considering whether I would date someone with a disability, the answer is "no." I can't imagine that as a possibility, especially if both of us needed attendant services. It would just be too weird. I want someone who is able-bodied and with whom I can have a relationship where the attendants aren't always around doing stuff for me. Not that I want my able-bodied lover to be my attendant, but just knowing that if in a pinch they were able to do something, like putting me to bed if we came back late from a date, then I wouldn't worry and would feel like my relationship with them was mine and not under scrutiny by others.

Partners may worry that our disabilities make us more fragile, and therefore might be reluctant to engage in certain activities or positions. They need to learn to trust us and our judgment about what is okay and what isn't. Sometimes our perceived problems can be an excuse not to do something when there is really another reason.

We also make assumptions about what partners might want or what they think. We might avoid suggesting something that we think wouldn't be that exciting for them. We may assume that they need to be protected from seeing our scars or dealing with ostomy bags or assistive devices. We need to check out these ideas and find out what our partners actually feel.

Well, there are sexual activities that I don't participate in anymore. Mostly, because I can't. I miss those activities a great deal and this impacts my self-esteem. It is much more difficult for me to help my partner to orgasm than it used to be. Now, I often wonder why would anyone want to have sex with me. My sex life mainly consists of my partner masturbating me and then masturbating herself with verbal encouragement from me. She has never wanted sex as much as I. So, sometimes (in fact, most times) she just masturbates me. I have noticed that we don't have sex as often as we used to, which worries me. I wonder whether the sex isn't any good anymore. This has been causing friction in our relationship in the last three or four years.

Uncertainty has contributed a lot of insecurity and a concomitant lessening of trust has sometimes created a less conducive atmos-

phere for sexual activities and trust—particularly in initiating sex. Fear of hurting (irrational) or exhausting me has also had its impact.

I'm not as physical. We now have to make love in ways so as to not hurt me. My partner is a very passionate lover and sometimes I think she has to hold back because she's afraid she might hurt me. Nothing can take the pleasure out of sex like a leg cramp. One of my favorite positions used to be on my knees but that is no longer an option. As my disease progresses we continue to experiment with new positions and sometimes find new and exciting ways to pleasure each other.

My current partner has also been encouraging, though we have our problems. She wants to have sex with me, and loves being eaten, but she often won't let me really do what I want to do because she's afraid of hurting me. She's constantly worrying about my wrist and finger pain if I fist her, even though that hurts a lot less than reaching inside her with a finger or two when she's bumping against my thigh. Since it hurts to hold myself up, I want her to be on top when I eat her, but sometimes she won't lower herself enough for me to really kiss her everywhere I want to or to get my tongue inside her. The best position for me, with her torso straight up, sitting on her ankles just over my mouth, we've only done once or twice because she's afraid of suffocating me. And though I want her to fuck me with our strap-on, it usually slips out if I'm on my back, and she's afraid that I'll hurt myself trying to stay up on my hands and knees. Sometimes we pile pillows under me, but I've noticed that she worries about my pain least when she's in a position that she likes, not a position that I like. I'm sure she's not consciously doing it, but she seems to be able to throw her concerns to the wind when she's having a great time, but not when I am. That makes me wonder whether the most important issue really is accommodating my disability or if it's accommodating her desire.

Get Involved and Get Outside

Difficult public transit, inaccessible buildings, and unwelcoming groups might make going out seem like more trouble than it's worth. But staying in leads to a downward spiral of isolation and loneliness. Getting involved in something politically meaningful is a safe and easy way to start getting out. Whether it's related to disability, gender, or something more overtly political, it's a chance to meet people who might enjoy doing other things together.

Other activities that are good for meeting people are volunteer work, musical groups, or hobby-related organizations.

Personal Ads and Dating Services

Many people have met partners through ads and dating services, though many others have been disappointed. Ads are often inexpensive and writing one is a good way to clarify what you are looking for. Look at other ads to get an idea of what people are looking for in different papers. Some papers have ads geared toward people looking just for sex, others more for relationships. When writing an ad, be honest. Don't say you are younger or older, taller or thinner, than you are. Don't pretend an interest or income you don't have. Remember when reading ads that not everyone is honest. When meeting someone through an ad, play it safe. Don't give your address. Arrange to meet in a public place at a time when lots of people will be around. You may even want to ask for references, friends who can vouch for the person.

> This dating service promised lots of dates, and I got them, but boy, most of the people they hooked me up with seemed to be the bottom of the barrel. We had nothing in common. A few of them weren't even looking for a relationship. They just wanted sex. I don't know if everyone who came to them was a loser or if they hooked me up with the losers because I have a disability and they thought that was all I deserved.

A good dating service will match up people who have the same interests or who seem likely to be compatible. Again, be honest. A dating service that has not had many clients with disabilities may think that they should only introduce people who have disabilities to each other, or that you will be grateful for any date they set up. You may want to address this issue with them before they match you up with anyone.

Finding People Online

Getting out isn't possible for everyone, but the Internet has given many people an opportunity to "get out" in a different way. The World Wide Web is a way to get information or become involved in a global community (whether a game-playing group, political organization, or hobby group), and is also a way that some people have sexual (or cybersexual) relations.

> *Go for it! (Though with just one full arm, I find it a bit tricky to type and self-stimulate at the same time!)*

> *I have much contact with people online. Sometimes I tell them I'm disabled; sometimes I don't. Many times they forget my limitations. Mental imagery really helps. I hope to meet one or two of the people I have chatted with next year. Whether we play or not, I'm undecided. I've also met people with whom I never discuss sex. One guy and I just play chess.*

Getting online is not something we can all do. Computers are expensive and so is adaptive software. Being sexual online requires access to a computer in a place where you can have some privacy. But the opportunity to communicate without sex and get information can be found at public libraries, community centers, and possibly your local center for independent living.

Relationships that start online can go almost anywhere. What you're looking for will greatly determine what you find. There are lots of opportunities for online sexual encounters, people who are looking for friends/pen pals, and people seeking long-term relationships through online dating services. Some people move the friendship or relationship to the real world, meeting in person. It is important to remember that when meeting someone online, they are not always who they say they are. If you are going to meet someone in person, you should arrange to meet them in public and with a friend around.

If you don't have one already, we highly recommend getting a free email address (from a service like Yahoo or Hotmail) and use that address for all your online explorations. While a computer hacker could find you anyway, most people wouldn't know how to track you down, and having a separate email address for when you go into chatrooms or email a personal ad gives you some anonymity and the ability to keep your primary email address free from unwanted junk mail.

Newsgroups, Dating Services, and Live Chats

Newsgroups are groups of people who subscribe to a list based on a common interest. Most often the group communicates through an email bulletin board where one member sends a message that gets sent to all the other members. There are newsgroups on practically every interest you can think of (sock knitters, people interested in the chemical properties of Play-Doh, fans of the original cast of "The Love Boat," not to mention every sexual interest under the sun). There are now several online sites that you can go to and browse through newsgroups to find a topic that interests you (see the Meeting People section of chapter 14). While the communications of the newsgroup are public, often relationships branch off into private communications. Meeting people is not the primary function of newsgroups, and some groups may be wary if you appear to be joining just to find a mate. When first checking out a newsgroup we recommend hanging back and reading some of the emails that the group is sending before venturing forth with your own email to the group. Some groups are filled with kind, interested people who are really there to support each other around whatever the group's subject interest is. But in most groups some people will be there primarily for an argument, wishing to pick on others and start verbal fights when they can. Surveying a group for a bit will give you a good idea of whom you might want to communicate with, and whom to stay away from.

Dozens of large, Internet dating services have proliferated, and hundreds of small ones. Among the benefits of these services is that they usually let you check them out for free, and also that concealing your disability (if you prefer to) is easier to do online. Most of these services offer you a mailbox, so you don't need to disclose your email address to the people you are responding to, or to the people responding to your ad. Every now and then an online dating service that is disability specific crops up. All our comments in the earlier dating service section apply here as well.

Chatrooms are Internet spaces, usually tied to a specific website, where people can communicate in real time. There will be chatrooms attached to websites with specific areas of interest (a website for a particular TV show might have a chatroom, or a political website might have a chatroom). Chatrooms also exist that are geared to sexual encounters. When you enter a chatroom you usually need to provide them with a name (never use your own!), but you can usually spend some time watching what is happening, reading what people are doing, before jumping in.

Another way of meeting people is to frequent disability-related sites that let you post personal ads. Sometimes these are free and sometimes they charge. If a site is going to charge you, try to get a referral from someone, find out if they actually have lots of people placing or answering ads, learn if the site has been around a while. Be wary of places that charge and be sure to get some information (and preferably a referral) before paying for stuff online. Some of the disability- and sex-specific sites listed in chapter 14 offer personal ads for free or for a minimal charge.

Paying for Sex

Some people say there's no such thing as free sex. We're not going to argue that position one way or the other, and we know that including information about prostitution will probably anger some folks. But the fact is that millions of people around the world, every kind of person you

DEVOTEES

Kath Duncan is a dynamic, fun, forty-something lesbian who works as a radio teacher and broadcaster, writer, and journalist in Australia. Born with one full-length right arm and one full-length left leg, she gets twice as much wear out of a pair of socks.

"Put simply, a devotee is someone who admires, desires, and/or fetishizes someone who's disabled. It can be any disability, but most common tend to be amputees, wheelchair users, and other physical or mobility disabilities.

"Opinions on devotees are very mixed within disability circles, with some claiming they are troubled, exploitative freaks who should be shunned. Others say they enjoy interacting with them, both as potential lovers or allies.

"The question really is: What does an attraction to physical difference mean? It's possible the attraction may not represent some bizarre problem, but may be just a variation on the big tits, red pubic hair, tight butt fetishes of other people, though we tend not to call these desires fetishes. We tend to class attractions as 'normal' and 'abnormal,' and an attraction to disabled folk is firmly assigned to the 'abnormal' basket. Restrictions on who we're supposed to be attracted to seem the only 'abnormal' thing to me. Maybe if disabled people on the whole weren't so excluded from life and 'normal' life experiences, then the devotee attraction would not seem weird at all, but rather a factor of the magical continuum of desire, or the notion that there's at least one somebody for everybody—and hopefully, in all our cases, lots of somebodies.

"Devotees say the disability is an 'attractant,' that is, a starting point for a relationship or an affair. There are sites on the Internet for several organizations that arrange group meetings between devotees and disabled individuals in a nonthreatening social environment." —KATH DUNCAN

can imagine, pay people for sex. It's not just for weirdoes, politicians, or televangelists. It can be for us, too.

We aren't suggesting that *anyone* has to pay for sex. People can live their entire lives without having sex with anyone (even themselves). While some people feel it's a necessity, it isn't exactly like oxygen. People pay for sex because they choose to—even if they feel they have no other place to get sex, it's still a choice. And some people who have no problem finding partners still choose to pay for sex. And we think that as long as both the client and the sex worker are doing everything consensually, sex work is not something to be put down, and sex workers should no longer be marginalized as evil, moral-robbing harlots. Sex work exists. It happens and people have access to it. People who are thinking of paying for sex need to think about how to access paid sex in a safe way, communicate what they want, and insist on safer sex practices.

We use the term *sex worker* as opposed to *prostitute*. *Sex worker* is a broader term that encompasses anyone who works in the sex industry. Someone who has sex for money and works off a street corner is a sex worker, so is someone who strips on the Internet and bills your credit card, so is someone doing phone sex for pay. The other thing we like about the term is that it is more descriptive of the fact that it's work. It's work that some people do by choice and other people do out of necessity.

All kinds of sex can be bought. Phone sex, sex online, strip clubs, massages to climax, oral sex, vaginal or anal penetration, and S/M sex are all available. If there is something you are interested in doing, it's likely that there is someone you can pay to do it with you.

Here are a few tips from sex workers themselves about communication beforehand and making sure you don't get ripped off.

Know what you want. The clearer you can be with someone about what you want *before* you start doing it, the better. If you're looking for someone to fuck, say so. If you want a specific kind of sex, let them know. Remember that it's their job and you are unlikely to shock someone with your sexual desires.

Have a safety plan. If you're having sex where you live, be aware that you could get robbed or hurt. Someone who will need help to defend themselves physically or to kick someone out should consider having someone at their place (obviously in another room), or should have a plan to call someone or have them call a couple of times during the visit. If they don't get the call, or if the phone isn't picked up at the appointed time, they'll know something's up and come over.

When possible get a referral. There are so many "escort" agencies in the yellow pages and personal ads in big-city newspapers that it's hard to tell who is good and who isn't. As a general rule, escort agencies in

SEXUAL SURROGATES

A sexual surrogate is someone trained to work with individuals to help them deal with sexual dysfunction or explore their sexuality.

Usually a surrogate will work with a therapist and a client. While traditional therapies usually focus on talking, a sexual surrogate will engage in sexual behaviors with the client, often using specific techniques that have been shown to be useful.

The goal of the encounter is to allow the client to explore aspects of sexual response, sexual feelings, and sexual techniques in a safe environment with a professional who is trained to provide feedback and offer suggestions and advice.

Sex surrogates usually charge about $100 an hour. Some surrogates may offer sliding-scale hourly rates. We are not aware of any health plans that cover the cost of sexual surrogates.

Despite the fact that surrogates have sex with you for money, surrogates distinguish what they do from prostitution because they have received specialized training and the main goal of the interaction is education. They are generally not treated like prostitutes by the law, and in most countries seeing a sexual surrogate is not something that will get you in legal trouble. It's a fair and important question, though, to ask about the legal status of someone you are considering working with.

Surrogates are not substitutes for finding dates or sexual partners; they are a step toward self–discovery, rather than a place to go just to have sex. Surrogacy is always a time-limited relationship. A sexual surrogate will agree to work with you for a set number of sessions, but will not offer open-ended therapy.

If you are interested in finding out more about sexual surrogates, contact the International Professional Surrogates Association, listed in the Sexuality: General Resources section of chapter 14.

Journalist Mark O'Brien wrote a marvelous article about his experiences with a sexual surrogate for *The Sun*. You can access the article online at www.pacificnews.org/marko/sex-surrogate.html.

the yellow pages should be avoided unless there is a specific recommendation from someone trustworthy. If you can't ask around, then insist on speaking with the person on the phone beforehand. Take this opportunity to do a little interview. Tell them about what you're looking for and ask them a few questions about their work. Ask them what they know about disability. Their responses will, we hope, give you an indication of what they are like to work with.

Talk about your disability. The last thing you need is someone either freaking out or throwing all their negative attitudes on you when you're supposed to be having fun. While you are having a relationship with a sex worker, you aren't friends, and you aren't going to be long-term lovers. Be up front about any assistance you need and whether or not you'll have an attendant there. If you'd prefer someone to assist you as part of the work, let them know. If you need time for positioning, you may want to find out if extra time will cost you more, or if they are comfortable with a slower pace.

Negotiating with Attendants

The topic of sexuality and attendants is a tricky one. We believe that sex and sexuality is an activity of daily living. Whether we are actually having sex or not, our sexuality is part and parcel of who we are, and an attendant has to deal with aspects of that, just like they have to deal with aspects of our race, religious faith, and food allergies. This doesn't mean that attendants have to deal with *all* aspects of the sexuality of their employers, just some. Your attendant may need time to adjust to this idea. It is an employment relationship and you have the right to expect it to be treated as such.

We can state categorically that sexuality is the most complicated thing attendants and their employers have to negotiate. We aren't suggesting that it's your job to make your attendant comfortable with the topic, or to pander to their issues about sex or morality. But the topic doesn't usually come up during an interview, and some tact is required in broaching the subject.

When we are talking about assistance, we are not talking about direct sexual contact between you and your attendant. We are referring to an attendant's facilitating sex play either for you on your own, or with someone else. They may be helping you set up a vibrator to play with, helping you put on a condom, or positioning you for sex with someone else.

Remember that you likely don't know anything about your attendant's sex life or beliefs. All of us are raised to think that everyone else has a better sex life and are much more comfortable with their own sexuality. Don't assume an attendant is more comfortable with sex than you are. Don't assume he or she has a good, healthy sex life. Don't assume anything. They may never have had sex, or their only sexual experiences could have been coercive ones, involving assault. They might be quite happy with their own sexuality and sex life but extremely uncomfortable discussing someone else's. When you bring up sex you may be pushing all sorts of buttons for them that they aren't prepared to have you push. They may also be anxious because you are their employer. While attendants often don't behave like employees, when they are put off guard (which is what talking about sex does to many of us) they may shift into a more submissive or defensive stance.

It isn't always best to launch right into asking how they feel about assisting with putting on a condom, or going to a strip club, or cleaning a vibrator. Of course you will know best, depending on the situation, but you may want to start a more general conversation about privacy and intimacy. If you think the attendant doesn't even see you as a sexual person, you could make it clear that you are, maybe by saying something like, "John is coming over and we'll probably have sex, so I'd like to have a bath first."

It may not always be easy or possible to talk with an attendant about getting assistance to express your sexuality. But that doesn't mean that exploring this is impossible. You will probably develop a sense from your working relationships with attendants as to who will be open to talking about this and who won't. You may be able to find other people who have been successful in negotiating this type of support from their attendants. You might be able to talk to them about what their experience was.

Unfortunately, some attendant service providers do not openly discuss this issue with staff or consumers, and assume that attendants and consumers will negotiate this without their involvement. As well, some attendants will not be open to even considering this as an extension of what they do in their jobs and, as a result, may have quite negative reactions to your desire to discuss or explore this with them. Be prepared for this. If you start making your wishes known, it is very possible that there are others who will also begin similar discussions.

Here are some practical suggestions from people who use attendant services:

- If you're thinking of having sex with someone else, start talking with the person you are interested in having sex with. If they are not knowledgeable about what attendant services mean (and what that might mean for you with regard to sex and sexuality), explain to them what you use your attendant for and the work relationship you have. Talk with this person about how the system works within your living situation. For example, if you have gender-specific attendants assisting with your personal care routine, how might your partner feel having either someone of the same sex or opposite sex assisting with positioning?

- Introduce your partner to your attendant and help them feel comfortable with each other. Talk to your partner about how she or he feels after meeting the attendant to see if they are comfortable with the process.

- Talk to your attendant about his or her comfort level in being able to provide support to you so that you can be sexual with yourself or with others. Not everyone is going to be cool with this, and this may be something they have never considered before. They might need to get more information. If possible, explore some resources for them so that they can find out about positive experiences people have had in using attendants.

- Talk to your attendant about what you're going to need them to do for you. Be as clear as you can about what type of assistance you need and what you do not need. Be open to talking about setting boundaries for yourself and the attendant. While the attendant is there to provide assistance, doing so may bring up personal concerns for them. They may want to discuss this with you or someone else. Explore with the attendant who else he or she might talk to about this. We know that talking openly about this kind of support is not something every attendant supports or is in favor of. Respect the attendant's need for privacy among other attendants (that is, don't pass on personal confidences to others).

Communicating with Health Care Professionals About Sex

I was in for my annual physical checkup, everything was fine and in working order. The doctor asked me if I had any other concerns or problems. Spelling on my letter board, I said, "Yes, there is just one thing." He cleared his voice in a rather impatient manner, and said, "Okay, what is it?" I explained that I was having some anxieties of a sexual nature. He took off his glasses and said in a stern voice, "I am only responsible for your health and well-being. If you'd like I can refer you to a counselor to talk about that stuff." I was left with the question, Isn't my sexual health related to my well-being as well? I then quickly realized what would also help in my health and well- being was to get another doctor.

It can be very hard to bring up sexual issues with a doctor. They are often rushed and may not give any easy openings into a conversation like this. You are left to ask about it out of any context. Doctors have a widely variable level of knowledge about sex. Some medical schools offer sexuality courses as electives, or give one lecture on sexual dysfunction as part of gynecology or urology courses. Others have a much fuller sexuality curriculum.

Before you go to the doctor, think about what you would like to discuss. Because doctors tend to interrupt patients early on when they are trying to tell their concerns, it is best that you prepare a question that is only one or two sentences. Then you can fill in the details. It is also helpful if you know the nonslang words for your sex organs and sexual functions (see chapter 3).

Doctors are required to keep communications with patients confidential, but that doesn't mean they always do this. It is a good idea to ask about confidentiality as a way to remind them that this is important to you. If you will have an attendant with you at the meeting, you can ask them to step outside while you are talking. If you will be using an

TIPS FROM AND FOR AAC USERS

For those of us who use augmentative or alternative ways to communicate (AAC), we offer a few tips that might be helpful when communicating important issues with our health care provider or others. One is to remember to bring our communication display or device to appointments. When communicating about issues related to our health or sexuality, it is helpful to have the vocabulary we need in our system or on our board to share our concerns. This includes words or pictures about body parts, feelings, medications, positioning, or possible questions.

It helps to have clear instructions on how we use our communication system. These instructions could be attached to the display or programmed into the device. The instructions should probably contain information about how we communicate and what we want speaking people to do when we are communicating with them. Some of us find it useful to have a "personal passport." This might contain information about how we communicate. For example, it might say, "I point to the picture I want to communicate using my index finger on my right hand." The passport can have instructions to the speaking person, such as, "Say the word out loud when I point to it, hold my display in front of me." We might include information about important things to know, like "Talk directly to me, not to the person who is with me, and give me time to communicate." Finally, the passport might contain key personal information; for example, "My name is…"or "In case of emergency call…."

One initiative called Speak Up has developed an excellent series of communication displays related to sexual health and pleasure. Speak Up is listed in the Sexuality: Disability-Specific Resources section of chapter 14.

interpreter or communications facilitator, you can discuss confidentiality with them beforehand.

At some point you just have to jump in and ask your question. Your doctor might feel as uncomfortable about hearing it as you do saying it, so if the response you get seems odd, this doesn't mean there is something weird about you or your question. You can also ask your doctor how much he or she knows about sex and your condition.

Exercises

1. Talk to someone (or yourself, out loud) about the last sexual dream or fantasy you had.

2. Ask a couple of people you know what they learned about their bodies and sex when they were young. If you have both nondisabled and disabled friends, do a comparison. Were they given words to use for penis, vagina, ass, anus, breasts, clitoris? It's a fascinating game to see how the words we're given (or not) are used to keep our behavior in line.

3. Make two lists of what you want out of sex. These lists aren't for anyone else, and you don't need to write them down. One list should have on it all the things you've ever fantasized about sexually. This may include things that you think are wrong or illegal, things you would never actually want to do in real life. The second list should be of things you would like to do, whether you've tried them before or not. Don't think about these lists as needing to be long, or needing to have any specific kind of behaviors on them (it's not a contest).

5

Sex with Ourselves

*Wanking is brilliant and always important!
Fortunately I know my own body best and so
am my own most proficient wanker!*

One of the most common questions we're asked when
we do workshops is how people living with certain kinds
of disabilities masturbate. How do quads masturbate?
How does someone without arms and legs masturbate?
How do people with severe arthritis masturbate?

Our first answer to this question is "That depends on
what turns them on." Right away, this moves us past the
assumption that everyone masturbates the same way,
because they don't. If masturbation is the act of self-
pleasuring, then we need to start with our minds, with
what gives us pleasure, not with functional considerations (such as "I want to rub my clit but can't reach"). So

we first figure out what gives us pleasure, what we find arousing, and from there we can begin to be creative about how we masturbate. Masturbation isn't just about genitals, or rubbing, or any of the other clichés we gather from TV, radio, the Internet, magazines, or pornography. It is solo sex. To emphasize this point many educators have dropped the clinical-sounding term *masturbation* and have replaced it with *solo sex* or *self-pleasuring*. We'll use all three alternately throughout this chapter.

Things to keep in mind about masturbation:

- You don't need to be naked to masturbate.
- You don't need to have an orgasm for it to be masturbation.
- You don't need to have all your nerves working to masturbate.
- You don't need to be able to reach or touch your genitals to mastur-bate.
- You don't need to do anything physical to yourself to masturbate.
- Masturbation is not second best to anything.
- All you need to masturbate is a plan and the energy to carry it out.

We also have to get rid of the idea of solo sex as a milestone, a goal that must be accomplished. This may not be possible, or may be possible only with help, and can be hard to achieve.

I would like to masturbate, but I've no one I feel comfortable with to ask for help.

Try not to add masturbation to the list of burdens in your life. Many people who cannot masturbate in the "traditional" ways end up feeling ashamed of it. If you are going to masturbate, do it for fun, relaxation, and emotional, psychological, and physical pleasure, not because you think you have to.

Masturbation has constituted 99.99 percent of my sex life. I never had a lover until 1995 and that didn't last long. I've been too embarrassed to ask for help. I can't use my hands at all, so I could use some help. When I was a teenager, I'd try to twist my body this way and that way so I could make my shorts tight. I'd lift my left knee, which is the only part of me that can move, and drop my thigh on my genitals. The pain turned me on terrifically. Now I can't lift my knee anymore. A friend once told me she was going to a sex toy store and did I want anything? I was dumbstruck. Why would I buy a sex toy if I couldn't use it? Or have a lover to help me use it?

If you acquired a disability later in life and masturbated one way before your disability, you may have to become willing to change your routine. Because masturbation is the first way most of us learn to be sexual, it often sticks as "the way" we get turned on, get aroused, and get off. In this way our masturbation routine can be a place to get stuck if we think there is only one way to do it. Luckily there's no age limit to learning new ways to masturbate.

Why Masturbate?

When I get off, I get to control the scene…who says and does what and when.

Many sex educators consider masturbation, however you practice it, to be the cornerstone of sexual health. Masturbation can be tangible proof that you can feel pleasure in your body or your mind and that you can be the instigator of that pleasure as well as in control of when and how the pleasure comes.

Self-pleasuring can be a political act that defies the idea that we get sexual pleasure only from certain kinds of sex. Self-pleasuring can also play a big role in improving body image. One of the hardest things about changing body image is combating all the negative messages we get about our bodies. "I look funny," "I'm too fat," "This part doesn't work right" are some thoughts that get in the way of our feeling good about ourselves. Negative messages can lead to hatred of our bodies. One of the ways to fight this is to start loving our bodies, as New Agey as this sounds ("love your body, use the force…"). Self-pleasuring is, literally, loving your body—telling it that it is worthy of pleasure, of positive attention, of a gentle (or rowdy) thought or touch.

Far from being second best, or the kind of sex people have when they can't have "real" sex, masturbation can be a tool for expanding sexual experience and knowledge. It is also the most frequently performed sex act in the world.

How can masturbation have such positive effects? First, it usually allows us to have a little more privacy than when we have sex with a partner. Having fewer distractions means we can focus more on our own feelings, how our body is responding and when. It means we won't be caught up in someone else's reactions or sexual agenda. Most people experience some form of performance anxiety when they are having sex with someone else. Thoughts about being good enough, attractive enough, saying the right thing, doing the right thing, smelling the right way, all serve to distract us from the point of having sex: feeling pleasure and experiencing our own responses and reactions (as well as that of others, if they are involved). So self-pleasuring may feel less pressured than other kinds of sex. When partners are involved we also give up a certain amount of control. Even if we can control our own body and responses, we don't know what the other person or persons will do. When we are alone, even if we use someone to assist in parts of it, we don't have as many unknowns. This is especially important if we don't know what to expect from our own sexual response—maybe because of a major change due to trauma, or if by chance we have never been sexual at all.

People who are able to have orgasms, but never have, often find that exploring their sexuality without a partner gives them the time, the control over the pace of the activity, and the ability to make adjustments in what they are doing that can lead to orgasm.

> *Masturbation is important to me. Times when I've felt too tired for partner sex, it is still comforting to masturbate. And before my current relationship, when my illness made it difficult to meet people, so that I thought I wouldn't find someone to date, I also took comfort in knowing that I could still masturbate. When I feel too sick to masturbate, I know I'm "really" feeling bad.*

I enjoy masturbation because I get "stressed" and do it to keep from making future relationship mistakes. I use a back-scratcher to reach because my disability limits my range of arm movements. I usually also do it when someone (caregiver or folks) thinks I am doing something else. I also take part in cybersex when I find some-one I feel is trustworthy.

When I first got hurt, masturbation was an issue. I would get an erection by fondling myself and jack off as hard and fast as I could. But every time I always ended up with a swelled penis and basi-cally hurting myself. Nothing happened, so it ended up being a joke that sometimes bothered me a hell of a lot. Mostly because an erection and jacking off at that stage of my life was important.

Hell, yes, I love it! First had an orgasm when I was about six or seven and became an expert by the age of twelve. Still masturbate now about twice a week and thoroughly enjoy floating off on my special sexual fantasies, usually about people I know.

Your Own Time

Privacy is something nondisabled people often take for granted. It can be very hard to access, though, when one is living with a disability or chronic illness. But private moments can still be carved out of most lives.

Even though I am often by myself, I never know when someone will walk in on me. I may look back and think, "I've just had half an hour to myself, I could have masturbated," but the time wasn't guaranteed. It isn't really my time.

Start by taking inventory of your privacy. If you live in a group home, boarding house, nursing home, or institution, or even if you rely on a pool of attendants whom your neighbors also rely on, chances are you have either no privacy at all or precious little. Look at your day and identify the times when you can count on being alone. Are there any workers who you think are enlightened enough to support your request for more privacy? If this isn't possible at first, consider the fact that as you fight for your rights others may begin to do so as well, and eventually you might get some results. If you are needing support or more information on advocating for your rights to privacy, contact your local center for independent living (see chapter 14 for contacts).

Even with all the privacy in the world, some people may still feel ashamed that they masturbate. They may have been taught as children that touching themselves makes them dirty, or may have been punished for touching themselves. Childhood trauma, such as sexual abuse or medical procedures to their genitals, can also make masturbation feel like a shameful act to some. We may also feel our bodies are not worth pleasuring because of the many negative messages we get from our disability-phobic society. So, when creating a private space, we can make an attempt not just to shut out the external world, but also to leave the shame out in the cold too.

Other people may have hours and hours alone, but have never set aside any of it as special time. They may spend much of their time by themselves feeling lonely and do not "seize the moment" for some private, quiet time. The important thing about private time is that it is intentional. Note the difference between time devoted to yourself, and time devoted to avoiding other things. Private time is time you set aside with the clear understanding with yourself that this time is for you to increase the pleasure in your life. Betty Dodson, the author of *Sex for One* (considered by many to be the masturbation "bible"), writes about how we constantly carve out specific time for other people, friends, family, even doctors, because doing things for others, or reporting to them, is considered important and worthy of devoting time to. Yet we rarely treat time alone with the same respect. One of Dodson's first instructions to improve your own sex life is to make a date with yourself—get excited about being alone and sexual with yourself as if it's a new thing. Treat solo sexual exploration with as much thought and respect as you treat exploration with a partner.

Time alone is also time you can devote to experience feelings in the parts of your body that don't cause you pain or discomfort. Because pain can be so overwhelming, you may only feel the pain, thus missing out on other, pleasurable sensations.

> When the pain from my occipital nerve flares it's like the rest of my body doesn't exist. My whole body changes to compensate for the pain (muscles tighten, posture shifts, even my facial expressions are different) and I usually don't realize this until after the pain has gone and all of the sudden I become aware of other parts of my body and of how sore they are.

Getting Started

> As a paraplegic, masturbation was a bit of a learning experience filled with trial and error. I have no sensation in my skin from the waist down, so masturbating the way most men do was simply not going to work for me. Over the years, starting in my teens I have discovered which parts of my body were sensitive to erotic touch and would help me to come to climax. My nipples are a very erogenous zone. I have also found the skin of my inner thighs, where I do have some sensation, is also a place I can touch and caress to give myself pleasure. Due to the nature of my disability I have not been able to ejaculate. I do, however, still experience the other sensations of orgasm. So I don't feel that the lack of ejaculation is that big of a deal.

We define *self-pleasuring* as any kind of sex play designed by you, that you initiate, where you are both the giver and receiver of pleasure. Having a sex fantasy in the middle of the day is masturbation. Having phone sex and getting turned on by the talk is masturbation. Having your attendant put a vibrator on (or near) you and leave the room so that you can play with it is masturbation. Going out and renting an adult video to watch, or streaming a scene to your computer, is masturbation. Arranging yourself just so in the bath or shower to have the water hit you where you like is masturbation. Sneaking off to the washroom at a meeting to jerk off is masturbation.

The first step is to find somewhere private and relax. If you don't have access to time alone, privacy might mean closing your eyes and pretending to be asleep. Start with relaxing your breathing, making it slow and steady, with a long exhalation. Your breathing will change with excitement, but you want to start relaxed. Try to remove any distractions (if you left the tap dripping, or forgot to take your meds, attend to it now, so that your mind isn't drawn back to it).

If you already have sexual fantasies or thoughts, here are some questions to ask yourself:

- What sparks my fantasies? Are there sounds, smells, sights, textures, or memories that take me into a fantasy?

When I want to get turned on there are some memories I go back to. The smell of the aftershave that a boyfriend used, the feeling of my hand on a guy's bum. Since I have very little vision, my fantasies are never about how someone looks. It's mainly my memories of how things have felt, and imagining things I haven't tried. But I can always get going with these thoughts.

- Are my fantasies vague or specific?
- What do I like to fantasize about?
- What am I wearing, and where am I?

I've always wanted to dress up in a really slutty outfit for sex. But all those things look like they would be difficult to manage with my arthritis. I do have some satin underwear that feels great, but I want more. So in my fantasies I have on one of those merry widow things. Sometimes I have a G-string on too, sometimes nothing else. I see myself looking in the mirror. Sometimes just imagining the look of that is all I need; other times there is another person in the fantasy telling me that I look like a slut and that I turn him on. Sometimes if I want to go really slowly I start all covered up with a robe or flannel pajamas and then slowly peel my clothes off.

- Is one sensation prominent in my fantasies?
- Am I alone or are there other people with me?

• What is everyone in the fantasy doing?

We can use fantasy alone as a way of self-pleasuring, and can take ideas from fantasies to try in other kinds of sex play.

Sometimes I like to masturbate when I feel stressed at work. I go to the wheelchair bathroom near my office to get off. I like to put my wheelchair facing the toilet bowl and then put one leg on the toilet seat, resting it against the grab bar. I move my bum toward the edge of the seat, lean back into the chair, and hike up my skirt. I usually start off with one fantasy that gets me hot pretty fast 'cause I only have so much time before getting back to my desk. I start rubbing my breasts through my bra until my nipples get hard. After I rub my nipples, I like to start rubbing my crotch on the outside of my underwear. When I am horny I notice a different kind of feeling in my body. My breathing gets faster and shallow and I get more excited at the thought that I could be heard by others outside of the washroom. When I come I feel my body totally relaxes but I also feel like I have more energy. I don't feel so stressed. When I masturbate at home, there is a different feeling because then I can take my time and focus on my whole body and how it feels but in the meantime, this does the trick.

If you haven't ever had a sexual fantasy, go ahead and set up a scenario. Imagine a place where you might feel sexual. Add in sounds, smells, or sights that might turn you on. Imagine what you are wearing, any sex toys you might want to have around. Then add in a sexual situation, either on your own or with another person or persons, and see where it goes.

What to Use

I started jerking off when I was living at the group home. I learned to do it quickly because I shared a room with another guy and didn't always have a lot of quiet time to myself. Now I live on my own and take all the time I need. On the weekends, I like to stay in bed late. I get the staff to help me lie on my side with a pillow between my legs. I have use of one hand and use the pillow as friction when I'm rubbing my penis. I like the changes in my body when I begin to breathe slow and then when it gets faster because I am getting hornier. My fantasies are about my girlfriend going down on me, and others are about her and me having sex with other people. Even though I like to take my time, sometimes I come really hard and fast. I think I come fast because when I lived in the group home I did not know when someone would come.

Before I got sick, my favorite way to masturbate was to put a rolled-up pillow between my thighs and squeeze rhythmically. The way I placed the pillow, it would put pressure on my whole crotch. Then I got sick and ended up paraplegic. I still have feeling all over. I've been searching around for a way to get the kind of orgasms I had before. With my fingers my orgasm is more just in my clit. I got a vibrator, but it seems too fast—I hardly have a chance to start breathing heavy before I come. I tried putting my pillow between my legs and pushing on it with my hand, but I couldn't get enough pressure going. But then I found a smaller pillow that is quite firm. I place it the same way and press on it with my hand. I like doing this while I have a small, egg-shaped vibrator in my vagina as far up as I can get it. It isn't exactly the same feeling, but I really like it. In my city the only store that sells sex toys that I would feel comfortable going to isn't accessible, so I ordered the vibrators on the Internet.

No rules govern what you can and can't use to masturbate. Some tools for masturbation include fantasy, hands and fingers, pillows or stuffed animals, feathers, sex toys, and water. Water can be used by directing a hose, spa jet, or shower massager at the genitals. Both men and women enjoy the feeling of a well-placed blast of water. It is important not to direct the water into the vagina or anus. People who use shower chairs can have an adapter welded on that will hold the hose so that it can be aimed at the right spot. Make sure you have a good shower curtain, especially if you are holding the hose yourself, as there is a tendency to drop it when coming and it will spray all over. More details are given in chapter 9, all about sex toys.

Finding Your Hot Spots

Now, masturbation consists of rubbing my chest, nipples in circular motions, rubbing underneath my balls in the crotch softly (sounds different, especially with no feeling), but there seems to be "buttons" that are pushed that makes my chest area feel good when I rub my crotch area. There is a relaxing, comfortable feeling that I get. I can't exactly explain why, but it is there. And most important is that it makes me feel good.

Remember the exercises in chapter 3, where we asked you to explore your whole body in whatever way you could, figuring out where you like to be touched and how? This is where you put what you learned into action.

There aren't any rules. You can try a variety of positions. You can fantasize without touching, touch without fantasizing, or do both together. You can go slow or fast. You don't have to have an orgasm, but it is fine to have orgasm as a goal too. Solo sex is like piano playing: The key thing is to practice, practice, practice.

If you are on a medication that decreases your interest in sex, or you have a condition that leaves you feeling tired most of the time, you can still masturbate. It is quite possible to get sexually excited even when you are lukewarm about the idea of masturbating. One might wonder, "Why masturbate if I don't feel like it?" We can be willing to do something without being really enthusiastic about it. Some people might masturbate without being really charged up about it because they want the relaxation that comes afterward, or to distract themselves from pain or worries, or just to see what it will be like.

I find I have different feelings in my body depending on the time of day. I used to often jerk off in the morning, because I would wake up with a hard-on. But it was always really rushed, because my attendant was coming and I didn't want to be caught in the act. But I did find that it got me energized, and I still do it a few times a week. Now I masturbate more at night. It means I've been going to sleep sticky, because I haven't gotten up the nerve to ask to have a washcloth left for me, but I like it because I go much slower and the orgasm seems to happen in more of my body. It isn't as much a big explosion. I fall asleep incredibly fast afterward.

Orgasm for people who live with spinal cord injuries (SCI) usually requires a much longer period of stimulation than it did before injury. The majority of people living with SCI report sexual satisfaction even if they do not experience orgasm. Women living with SCI may find that stimulation of the cervix may increase their chance of having an orgasm. It can be difficult to reach the cervix with a finger, so a sex toy might be of help (see chapter 9).

Solo Sex with Others

Intercourse is painful and difficult for me, so we avoid it. We do all kinds of other stuff. I love having him watch me masturbate and also watching him masturbate. Sometimes one of us will tell a sexy story at the same time.

Masturbation is not always a solitary pursuit. Although we encourage everyone to start by themselves, so that they have the privacy to experiment, figure things out, and have sexual time that is all theirs, masturbation can also be very pleasurable as a shared activity. It can be a way to show your partner what you like, as well as learn what *they* like. Watching and being watched can be a real turn-on. Some women like to masturbate during intercourse. For others, it is a way to deal with one partner's fatigue.

Yes, yes, yes, I love masturbation! It was truly my greatest fear as an adolescent that I wouldn't have a sex life at all, and it was the greatest gift of my life to realize this was not the case. Through my sexual relationships I have learnt more about myself and my attitudes to my body and done more self-healing than in any other area of my life. As far as this changing over time...well, no, if anything my love for my sexual expression has become more intense and more important than it was when I was fourteen, when its intensity filled my universe. I hope to remain an intensely, sexually exploring woman for all my life.

The Basic "How-To's" of Masturbation

There is no right or wrong way to masturbate. Because we're all different, it's hard to suggest specific techniques that will work for you. But here are some pointers to keep in mind:

1. Keep it wet. Use lots of lubricant, spit, or water. Almost everything feels better when it's slick and slippery.

2. Know your body. If you haven't already, we encourage you to go back now to chapter 3 and try out some of the exercises. They are intended to help you get to know your body. You need to figure out what feels good where. If you love having your neck rubbed, then make that the focus of your next masturbation session. If it's your clitoris or nipples that drive you wild, go for it.

3. Mix up the sensation. Sexual pleasure can come from friction (rubbing), vibrations, pressure, heat, or cold. Pressure can be applied with fingers, pillows, chair arms, stuffed animals, crutches, anything. Vibration can come from a vibrator, a shaking alarm clock, pulsating shower massager, or the edge of a washing machine. Try different kinds of feelings: pressing against something feels very different than hitting a part of your body, or lightly tickling it with a feather.

4. Penetration or external stimulation? People use either or both when they masturbate. Penetration can be with fingers, dildos and harnesses, or household objects (see chapter 9). You can turn yourself on externally by squeezing your thighs, positioning yourself in a particular way, or any of the ideas listed above (using water in the bath-

tub or shower seemed a particularly popular idea from our survey respondents).

One of the hardest things about creative masturbation is that so few people talk about it, making it challenging to learn from others' experiences. There are two websites devoted to masturbation, one for women, www.clitical.com, and one for men, www.jackinworld.com. Check out these sites for other tips and masturbation discussion, and if you've found a great way to get yourself off, write in and share your discoveries.

Sex with Others

We all go through stages when we are more interested in sex with others, or less interested. Sometimes we want to be sexual with someone because we feel an intense spark of erotic attraction for them. Or we may love them and want to *make* love to them. At other times we just itch to have sex—even though at the moment we may not glimpse a potential partner on the horizon. Whenever we find ourselves in sexual situations, we can enhance our pleasure if we communicate well with our partner, understand our own expectations, get down and dirty at the right time for us, and deal with anxieties that may arise during sex.

Communication

We've written a whole chapter about communication (chapter 4), but in case you skipped it to get to the "good stuff," we will just mention again that good communication is a key to good sex.

> *Once my husband and I had great sex just after I bought a low cut top and wore it with a push-up bra. Now, when I want sex and don't feel like I can just say it, I put on that bra and top. He'll walk into the room and see me and I can see he's getting an erection because he knows what I want, which gets me even more turned on.*

Good communication won't necessarily happen on the first date. While some people find it exciting to have sex soon after meeting someone, most people find that sex works better if they have developed ways of communicating first.

Devices that we use for communication may be inadequate for communicating about sex, and it can take some courage to ask to have your computer programmed with sex words, or a special Bliss board made with this vocabulary in mind. Many people communicate visually while having sex, which is helpful if you can't use words, but a challenge to people who are visually impaired. There are nonverbal, nonvisual ways of communicating what you are feeling and what you want. Touch can be used spontaneously, and by asking for it ahead of time, you can agree that touching certain parts of your partner means "Yes, yes, go on," while touching other parts means "No, this isn't doing it for me at all." You can also alternate pressure, so that a light touch may mean that what's going on is nice and a firm touch means that you want more *now*. If you haven't arranged signals beforehand, you can just put your hand over your partner's and guide it to where you want, then indicate what kind of pressure you want used.

Anxiety

People worry about sex. We worry about whether we will be able to figure out what to do. We worry about how we look. We worry about being rejected. We worry about having an asthma attack, stroke, or heart attack during sex. We worry that our disability will stop us from doing something we want to do.

All of this anxiety can decrease our pleasure in sex play (hey, now you can worry about that, too!). What will help with this is reassuring yourself that you will be able to figure it out, that your partner is interested in who you are, how you smell and feel and taste rather than how you look. Deep, slow breathing can also help if you are getting really anxious.

Some of the things that happen during sex are the same things that happen with anxiety—raised heart rate, sweating, fast breathing—and people who have had panic attacks may be worried that they are getting an attack. These symptoms (especially shallow, quick breathing) are also similar to some asthma symptoms and can cause similar worries. People living with asthma who think these feelings are from asthma, not excitement, can slow down, have a puff or two of medication, and use pillows to keep the chest and head elevated.

Expectations

If we think there is a certain way that we must have sex, or an outcome that is essential for satisfaction, then we are missing opportunities for enjoyment, expression, and increased self-knowledge. Our needs change over time, with age, changing levels of disability, and maturity. We can accommodate these changing needs by being open to a variety of experiences and outcomes.

> It is spontaneous each time. I used to get stuck, needing orgasm, needing penetration, etc. Now, my sexuality has matured to a place that experimentation and spontaneity make sex rich. For example, one of the greatest highs I get (full-body orgasms? or spiritual-like orgasms?) is from having my neck bit, though I have sensation over my whole body.

Timing

When I feel good I'm a very sexual person, but when I hurt I feel like sex is a chore and not a pleasure. When I feel good I see myself as a playful partner. I feel good about being with someone, but on the days the pain is worse I don't want to be touched. And that's sometimes hard for my partner to understand. Sometimes she thinks I'm mad at her. As my disease progresses I feel less sexual, but that doesn't mean I'm not still interested, just that my partner has to sometimes wait till I feel like sex.

Timing is always important. There are very few people who are always eager to have sex. We need to do other things in life, like sleeping and eating and going to work or to the park. Times of stress are often times when people don't want to have sex, although some people find sex to be a way to relieve stress. Letting your partner know some general guidelines about when you might be interested in sex can be helpful. You can tell them if there is a time of day when you are more interested, or at which times in your menstrual cycle. Unless you speak up it may not be otherwise apparent that you hate having sex when you are tired or in pain.

Try to pay attention to timing messages from a partner. If you don't pick up on these messages, you may end up feeling rejected when your offers of sex are turned down, merely because it is a less auspicious time for them to have sex.

Spontaneity

Successful spontaneity often happens as a result of careful planning. This may seem contradictory, but totally spontaneous sex is often disappointing and can even be dangerous. The idea that sex should be unplanned has led to numerous unwanted pregnancies, sexually transmitted infections, hurt feelings, and unsatisfying encounters. When we figure out in advance what we need to be safe and enjoy ourselves, and then communicate it to our partners, we have developed a framework within which there is infinite possibility. People tend to see this need for planning as a negative thing, but it is really an opportunity to expand our sexual horizons. Regardless of disability it can be a good idea to plan ahead for sex.

> In the past my sex life consisted of going to a bathhouse, making my way to a dark room, or the sauna without my wheelchair. I would get another man off by giving him head or jerking him off. However, this kind of sex was mostly one-sided. My partner got off.

> When I broke my neck at twelve, I never thought about sex, and rehab hospitals never even mentioned it to married couples for another eight to ten years. I have surgical scars all over my body and no muscle tone, so I look flabby. Plus, sex tends to be sponta-neous, but when disability comes, spontaneity goes. It's gotten worse as the number of surgeries have increased.

Energy

> Because my energy is so limited, usually having sex means choosing not to do some other activity later in the day. For instance, if we fool around on a Saturday morning, I can't get out of bed and go out to brunch afterward, and I may or may not be able to go to a movie that night. I have to rest. Also, I often want to fool around even when I'm feeling very exhausted. So sometimes we choose to have what I call "tired sex," where I do less, am less active, and have to be lying down all the time. With "tired sex" it can be difficult to get turned on—touching feels good at the specific spot being stimulated, but the pleasure doesn't spread to a more global escalation of excitement. And it can be hard to come if I'm very exhausted, even if I think I feel turned on. Even when I'm feeling energetic enough to have more

active sex, I'm restricted to less-strenuous positions—I can't stand up, I can't take weight on my arms, etc.

People living with lupus, kidney failure, arthritis, heart disease, and other chronic conditions may get tired easily and may be too fatigued to be interested in sex or to put any interest into action. Figuring out priorities becomes important. On certain days it becomes more important to get the grocery shopping done than to have sex, but on another day this might be reversed.

If you seem to have less energy than usual for sex, you might want to figure out why this is happening. Is your condition worsening? Are you getting less exercise? Are there problems in your relationship? Have your medications changed? Are you feeling depressed?

One of the problems with low energy is that a partner may assume that your claim that you're too tired to have sex really means you're not interested in them sexually. Partners will typically want to be reassured about this, and more than once.

When energy is low, you may be feeling sexual yet not notice. The cues may be much more subtle. You have to learn what these signals are, and to notice them when they occur. You then decide whether to act on them.

In addition to planning sex for times when you expect to have more energy, another helpful technique is the "stop and start." Start whatever sexual activity you are interested in, and take a break when you notice that you are getting tired. This break can be a complete rest, or can involve a less-strenuous activity. Start again when you have gathered some energy. This pacing can also introduce more variety into sex play and teasingly delay orgasm.

Sometimes people worry that their low energy is a sign that having sex would be damaging to them. Many people with heart disease hold this belief. If you can walk up two flights of stairs without chest pain, then you can safely have sex and should have enough energy to do so. An exercise program (with the guidance of a physical therapist or physician) can increase stamina and decrease both chest pain and shortness of breath during sex. Either of these symptoms, or having palpitations, is a signal to stop exerting yourself. Sexual activities that require little or no exertion, with you positioned on your side or back, lessen the chance of symptoms. Go slow in the beginning to minimize stress and fear of a heart attack.

Any illness that is associated with anemia can lead to decreased energy and interest in sex.

> When I was having dialysis three days a week, I would sometimes feel like having sex the night after a dialysis day, but never the next day. Now that I am dialysed six nights a week, I find my interest is a lot higher, but then timing is a problem. Sometimes I get unhooked from everything in the morning and then we "do it." I have also had problems keeping my erections.

Where to Have Sex

Finding a place to privately have sex can be a challenge, as discussed at length in chapter 4. People who have their own house or apartment, or whose partners do, have more choice about where to have sex. Those of us who live in group or shared accommodations have decreased options, and those in institutional settings have very limited choice. Flirting and verbal play can take place in public settings without anyone knowing what is going on, and sometimes spaces that are unused at certain times of the day can be utilized, like laundry rooms or service elevators.

People have sex in many places other than in bed. Floors, sofas, chairs, bathtubs, parks, and cars have all been turned into lovebirds' nests. Some of the more romantic-sounding settings, though, lose their charm when actually tried—sex on the beach sounds great until you get sand in your vagina.

> Accessible toilets are FAB.... One can get pushed in there by a lover and everyone thinks "Isn't that sad, someone needs to wipe their bum," and you can shag away in private and then come out

and no one has a clue as to what really went on! It's liberating and definitely one of the few perks of being a wheelchair user!

Fantasy

You might be surprised to learn that fantasy is not just a solitary experience. People incorporate fantasy into their sexual relationships first by having fantasies, then by sharing and creating them together (we talk more about this in chapter 11). People may have fantasies about things they like to do, things they would like to do but can't, and things that excite them even though they wouldn't want to try them.

One of our fantasies involves going to bed with another couple. We both believe that it is important not to feel guilty when engaged in this form of sexual play. Since I am disabled and my wife is able body, we usually like to pretend that the other couple would be complementary to our own situation: meaning that the woman is a paraplegic, like me, and the male is able body, like my wife. This fantasy allows us to think of other sexual possibilities that the limitations of our own bodies will not allow us to experience. In my own particular case, it allows me to compensate for my inability to reach an orgasm and ejaculate. I can then contemplate sexual intercourse in a more natural and a more spontaneous fashion, where there is arousal, erection, penetration, and ejaculation. This fantasy play lets me feel like I am a more complete sexual person. And I feel content with my sexuality. But it took me a long time to reach this point of contentment.

I tell my partner that I would like to tell her a bedtime story, and then I tell her a fantasy that involves the two of us. I do it like a story, so I start with "Once upon a time." Sometime I'll use "I" and "we," so it would be like, "I was on my way home and I saw some really sexy underwear in a store window. I told the paratransit driver that I wanted to stop and buy some and he stopped and said to take my time..." (The great thing about fantasy is that you can make things happen that would never occur in real life!). Sometimes I use our names, instead. "Joe bought the red lacy thong and slipped it into his pocket. When he got home, he said to Lily, 'I have a little surprise for you in my pocket, but you have to guess what it is.' " A couple of minutes into the fantasy she will start to masturbate or to touch me, and I just keep going on with the story for as long as I can.

One night we got a bit drunk and Susie dared me to tell her one of my fantasies. So I told her one of my favorites, where she and I are having sex and then I realize that there is someone watching us. She talks to the guy about how she's feeling, what she thinks he's thinking, what he'd like to be doing with us. We both got really turned on and started having sex and then she pretended my fantasy was really happening, pretended the guy was there. It was wonderful. Now we both share our fantasies. Sometimes if I don't have much energy, I'll tell her a fantasy and she'll masturbate.

Sharing fantasies with a partner can increase our comfort level with each other and add some variation to sex play. Sometimes people think there is something wrong with fantasizing about other people or scenarios during sex play. While people who have a tendency to "check out" during sex because of early trauma may want to watch this, having daydreams or fantasies while you're having sex with someone else doesn't have to mean you aren't interested in your partner. It may be a safe way of incorporating something into your sex life that you don't want to fully act out. A good example of this kind of fantasy play is sometimes called gender play.

Gender Play

I identify myself as bisexual, but I've never had sex with a man, unless you count the somewhat accidental jerk-offs that occur during personal care. I used to dress up. One of my attendants liked to dress up and he got me undies and wigs. When my black lace panties arrived in the mail, he put them on me. While putting them on me, he asked why I was groaning. I told him I was coming.

Gender play is based on the traditional gender roles we all live with (whether we like them or not, or accept them or not). These traditional roles say men must be aggressive, active, always on top, while women must be passive, the receivers, always trying to please the man. When it comes to sex, *gender play* refers to messing with the gender roles you are traditionally assigned. So if you identify as a woman, and you have a woman's body parts, gender play might mean going out and buying a harness and strap-on dildo and wearing it to bed. You might use it to penetrate your partner, you might have your partner go down on you (and your dildo), or it may just be there to let you get more fully into the role of a man. If you identify as a man, gender play might mean acting more like what you think a woman is. This might include getting dressed up, talking in a different voice, acting and touching your partner differently, or it could be something that is strictly in your head. Gender play is a form of fantasy, sometimes just in your head, and other times acted out. Within the safety of play with a sex partner we can give ourselves the freedom to explore other ways of being sexual, free of rules about how men and women are supposed to act or feel. There is a lot more written on this topic, and if you are interested in learning more you can check out the Gender, Queer, and Transsexual/Transgender Resources section of chapter 14.

Touch

Ashley Montegue has written about the importance of touch, that the many nerve endings in our skin crave to be stroked, caressed, and held. We could all survive without touch, but at a huge cost. Many of us have conflicting feelings about being touched. We may have been touched in ways we didn't like. We may have been touched without our consent. Touch may be associated with pain or betrayal. The good news is that the right kinds of touch can help us overcome these feelings. Sometimes it is helpful to start with professional touch—massage, Shiatsu, reflexology—and to work up to touch with a partner. Sexual touch includes a broad range of activities. It can be hair brushing, stroking a face, massaging feet, touching genitals. We learn about our partners through touch. We communicate about ourselves by the way we touch. Touch often starts *before* what we would traditionally call sex.

"Accidentally" brushing against a date's body, holding hands, running your hands through a friend's hair, placing a hand on a back or an arm during a conversation—all are tantalizing acts that can lead to sex. Sex starts with communication by way of words, touch, and nonverbal language. Too often, we don't value touch that doesn't lead to penetration. We rush through the "foreplay" to get to what we think is the real stuff of sex. Whether you are nervous about having sex with someone for the first time, or in a relationship where you feel the sex has gotten routine and dull, playing with touch (and not planning to have penetration) can be a great way to open up possibilities beyond what you expect. It's fun to get creative with touching. Touching can be as much about the intention and focus of the people involved as the physical sensation. Even if you lack sensation you can be turned on by touching someone or having someone touch you. If you aren't able to touch someone, you can still use touch by instructing your partner to touch themselves in ways that you describe to them. It may be their hand touching, but it's your mind that is guiding it. You may also be able to adapt your usual assistive devices for touching, by adding a piece of soft fabric, a feather, a scrap of leather, or a small stuffed animal. By discussing what will and won't work, you can probably figure out a way to make happen the kind of touch you want.

Orgasm

Because in my early sex life I felt so fearful, anxious, pressured, unable to say what I wanted, etc., I didn't have orgasms with other people. So now that I can have orgasms with my lover, it feels important to me that I do. However, neither my lover nor I feel that we have to have an orgasm every time we have sex. We also don't feel we have to have intercourse/penetration when we have sex, or that we even have to have sex when we've been making out or cuddling.

I come fairly readily with gentle clitoral stimulation—have never come through vaginal penetration with a penis no matter how skilled my lover, although I have come through someone's fingers sort of wriggling away inside me. I love coming—regard it as the high point of the whole event and would feel rather ripped off if I didn't come.

One of the most common expectations about sex is that both people will have orgasms. Some even expect that those orgasms will occur at the same moment. Orgasms can be wonderful, but sex without orgasm can also be terrific. We can get so focused on the goal of orgasm that we lose the joy of the sexual experience. We also tend to blame ourselves and feel incompetent if we have decided that orgasm is the most important thing and then are unable to attain it.

Some people have an orgasm in only one way—by having a certain part of them stimulated in a certain way—while others find they can have orgasms from more than one area or kind of stimulation. Some people learn to have orgasms from mental stimulation alone.

Orgasm can become a source of uncommunicated conflict in a relationship. If one or both people are blaming themselves (saying or thinking "I don't come fast enough," "I come too soon," "It's my fault I don't have orgasms," "We should come at the same time"), then it can become difficult to discuss the issue. If a discussion can start with the assumption that sometimes people have orgasms, and sometimes they don't, it is easier to move on to talking about what each person would like to have happen, how they think this could be achieved, things they would like to try. Not everyone has to discuss orgasm with every partner. It isn't always necessary, and besides that, sometimes it might not feel safe.

THE PHANTOM ORGASM

Traditionally, research about things like orgasm and disability has been carried out by nondisabled researchers. This has led to many problems in the way they choose to redefine what their test subjects report. An excellent example of the way information gets twisted is the term *phantom orgasm*. This was a term that researchers came up with to describe something their subjects reported. In early research with people with complete spinal cord injuries, some people would report having the feeling of an orgasm, despite not having genital sensation. The "expert" explanation was that these people were merely experiencing a body memory of an orgasm they knew before their injury. These orgasms were called "phantom," like ghost orgasms that hang around in our body waiting for the opportunity to trick us into thinking we are feeling something. Of course this kind of definition is more about narrow-mindedness of the researchers than what was actually happening. More recent research conducted by Beverley Whipple and her colleagues has shown that in fact women with complete spinal cord injuries do experience orgasm, sometimes from stimulation and sometimes from fantasy alone, and that these orgasms are not of lesser quality than other orgasms.

Orgasm is important, going back to its being in the mind, that if the person I am with shows their appreciation, orgasm and etc., I get off mentally, so it is important to know that they are enjoying themselves and release their feelings. I even have had orgasms from a woman and man, separately, when they have nibbled and sucked on my chest and nipple area, especially around the line of feeling. It sounds crazy, but there is this feeling that just releases a tingle through my upper body.

As my kidney failure got worse, I stopped having orgasms. My husband thought he was doing something wrong. Now, a year after transplant, my orgasms are back on track. No one ever warned me about this and I was too embarrassed to ask about it.

In addition to causing difficulties in getting sexually excited and having orgasms, kidney disease may decrease vaginal lubrication. Women's periods may stop and then start again with dialysis. These resumed periods may be longer and more painful.

Decreased lubrication can be a problem for women living with a number of chronic illnesses or disabilities, as well as a side effect of certain medications. Some women find it difficult to talk with their partners about this, as they feel lack of lubrication is a sign that they aren't excited enough. But this is often not the case, and lack of lubrication may be completely unrelated to how turned on you are. A wide range of water-based lubricants is available to provide a relatively inexpensive way to make penetration play more comfortable and arousing (see chapter 9 for more information on choosing the right lubricant).

Kidney disease, diabetes, other endocrine problems, and some medications (including antidepressants) can all lead to difficulties attaining orgasm. Some (but unfortunately not all) doctors feel comfortable bringing this up.

Orgasm is a total body experience. When a person comes, they experience a rapid heart rate and breathing, flushed skin, swelling of the head of the penis or clitoris, and a feeling of tension and release. Men can have orgasms without ejaculation. Ejaculation is not as common in women but is something many women experience, and can learn to do as well. (see our discussion of the G-spot in chapter 3).

> *Orgasm. Phew. Well, it is important to me at times, but it has not always been particularly enjoyable. The truth is that orgasm is most important to me if I am sore and wanting to sleep. I masturbate to help fall asleep once a week or more. During sex with a partner, I am very rarely looking to come. More often, I want to give my partner an orgasm. This is out of a history of bad sexual choices and surviving sexual assault and rape, not out of something related to my disability. My disability does have an effect, of course, but I'd already backed away from seeing orgasm as important before I ever identified as disabled. Acknowledging how my body is changing to tolerate less stress or use was most important in learning that my goals can change from minute to minute during sex. This didn't*

deemphasize orgasm, but it did give me more fluidity during sex.... In the past six months I have had some incredible orgasms. And now that I've given myself permission to change what I want in the middle of sex, I find that even though I rarely start sex with the goal of cumming, halfway through, if my partner touches me just right, I can find myself completely changing from being focused on pleasuring her to being focused on having my own orgasm, my way. I think it's fair to say that I rarely know what my goals are till I'm already deep into the sex my partner and I are having.

Fetishes

Very strong preferences for certain kinds of stimuli are called *fetishes*. In the medical system, fetishes are seen as sick or "aberrant" sexual behavior. However, most fetishes are not a harmful or dangerous aspect of the sex lives of people who experience them. For some people having a particular fetish means that it is the only way they can become sexually aroused. As long as the fetish doesn't involve hurting themselves, or somebody else, and is consensual, we don't think people should be quick to judge fetishes as abnormal or threatening.

Fetishes often involve objects. The term was originally associated with objects used in religious worship that were thought to have important, even magical, powers. A fetish object is something that elicits a strong sexual response from someone. It might be an article of clothing (shoes, boxer shorts, glasses) or a material (leather, silk). We can also fetishize particular scenarios, or types of people, or body parts, or skin colors.

Some people fetishize disabled bodies, and others fetishize the idea of disability as well (see sidebar in chapter 4). The most common theory about fetishes is that they stem from childhood experiences in which we associate an object or experience with a feeling. This feeling may have been sexual, or could have been a feeling of comfort or excitement. Perhaps someone was wrapped in a satin blanket the first time they masturbated and now they associate the feel of satin with sexual pleasure. There is no conclusive evidence about this, and anyway it doesn't really matter what causes it. Fetishes, like so much else, can either enrich or trap people. It tends to trap them when they feel they have an awful secret that they must hide.

Here are some common fetishes:

- A willing exchange of power with one person dominating the other is called S/M and is discussed in detail in chapter 11.
- Getting aroused by dressing up as the opposite gender is called transvestism. This is different from feeling you are really of the opposite gender, or wishing you were. Transvestites (also called *cross-dressers*) simply love the experience of dressing up and find it a turn-on.
- Exhibitionists get aroused by exposing themselves sexually in public. The classic example of this is a flasher who is turned on by exposing his naked body to unsuspecting people. (This particular act is clearly not consensual and is illegal in most places.) Exhibitionism can also be wanting to be sexual with someone else in public.
- When someone is aroused by looking at someone naked or watching them being sexual with themselves or others, they are called *voyeurs*.

There are countless other fetishes: *frotteurism* refers to getting turned on by rubbing against strangers (again, not a consensual activity); *pony play* is a fetish that involves one person dressing up as a "pony" and another person being the "rider" and riding them around. Numerous fetishes focus on body parts or hair. Foot fetishes seem to be the most common, judging by the number of magazines and videos devoted to them.

Additional Considerations for Sex with Others

Your sex with others will be more enjoyable if you have first thought through any particular challenges you have to deal with regularly, such as mobility and sensation concerns, tendency to spasm, incontinence issues, ostomy bag use, and hypersensitivity to touch.

Mobility and Sensation

When thinking about having sex, especially with other people, mobility and sensation are obvious considerations. It can be hard to feel sexy and to let yourself be sexual if concerns in these two areas are worrying you. Mobility has an effect on achieving pleasurable positions, nonverbal communication, and sexual safety. Individual variations in sensation need to be communicated to partners, which can be a challenge. The body-mapping exercise in chapter 3 can be used with a partner to help them understand where you have sensation and what kind of sensation you experience. You can also use it on them. There is a lot of variation in what parts of the body feel sexual. Often people just try to figure out where and how their partners like to be touched over time, but a body-mapping exercise can speed up the process—plus it can be lots of fun!

Much of what has been written about sex and disability deals with mobility and sensation, assuming that the primary question any disabled person would have is "How I can do *this* if I can't do *that?*" When reading the surveys that we based this book on, we were struck by how infrequently people addressed mobility and sensation issues. They are important issues, but our respondents were telling us that their biggest issue was getting over the hurdle of feeling sexy and letting themselves be sexual. Once they embraced their sexuality, they told us, figuring out how to have sex wasn't as hard as they had thought.

Our discussion of positions in chapter 8 addresses mobility issues. Dealing with mobility involves talking with partners about what you want to do and how you are going to do it. Mutual problem solving can be a fun exercise too, as you practice using toys, pillows, or any other props that you think may be useful or fun. Experimentation and creativity are equally important when dealing with sensation. Different parts of your body will have different sensation. Pleasure may be derived from what seem to be unlikely spots. Sensation can change over time, so remember to check things out regularly.

Spasticity

Feeling sexy is a challenge. I tend to tighten up during sex, so it makes it difficult to enjoy because I fear I may go into a flexer spasm.

I'm a big woman and my husband is a little guy. One night we were having sex and I started to spasm and trapped him between my thighs. He couldn't get out. I guess we could have waited it out but we kind of panicked and called 911. It was pretty funny, really.

Spasticity during sex can be a real challenge, especially as sexual arousal can bring on spasms. It can occur with CP, ALS, spinal cord injuries, and other neurological conditions. Bathing in warm water before sex may reduce spasticity, as well as relax muscles and joints. The bath can be incorporated into sex play. Some people take extra medication for spasticity before sex. If you are thinking of doing this, you may want to ask your health care provider about whether this is okay and when to take it. The relaxing effects of sex play may have the bonus effect of helping to reduce spasticity, so if spasticity is a problem for penetration, and penetration is desired, it can come later on in sex play. For women with hip adductor spasticity, rear vaginal entry lets the legs stay together while allowing penetration.

For men who can't straighten their legs, a good position is with the man on his back, his partner sitting on top. His partner can lean back against his bent legs. If his legs are right up against his belly, the partner can sometimes straddle the man on top of his legs, which allows for partial penetration.

The strategic use of pillows to prop legs into a comfortable position can help, especially when there are knee or hip contractures.

Surprise: Some people use spasms in sex. If your hand spasms, your partner may love to have it rubbed up against a part of their body that's very sensitive (say, their clitoris).

Some women with cerebral palsy (CP) have vaginal muscle spasms, interfering with penetration and causing pain. Avoiding penetration is one way around this. Some women find that the spasms go away after orgasm, so having an orgasm before penetration is another possibility.

Spasticity in the hands can make it difficult to put on a condom or insert spermicidal foam or a diaphragm. The E-Z On condom may be easier to put on, but is currently quite expensive (see chapter 12).

SHAME AND SILENCE

In an excellent article in *The Ragged Edge* called "It Ain't Exactly Sexy," Cheryl Marie Wade writes about the difference between those of us who can use the bathroom ourselves and those who can't. She points out the fundamental difference between these groups. The second group has much less privacy—as she puts it, "no place in our bodies (other than our imaginations) that is private." She also points out that few of us ever discuss this. The disability movement, along with the rest of the world, is always ready to emphasize the abilities, the importance of independence, which serves to remind us that if we require assistance with aspects of our daily living it says something about us; that we are less than; that we are broken. We all like to keep things neat and tidy, everything looking as "sexy" and "whole" as possible.

One way to start breaking this cycle is by explicitly talking about the "dirty" things in our lives. If we can begin by being proud of our ability to take care of ourselves, which may require extreme patience with letting others come into our most personal and private spaces, then we will be in a better position to begin these discussions.

Incontinence

Let's face it: Sex is a pretty wet experience, given female lubrication and both male and female ejaculation. Urinary incontinence can make it wetter, though not always noticeably so. Sexual stimulation can increase the chance of incontinence, but a regular bowel and bladder routine can minimize it. If there is a time of day that you are more likely to have sex, plan your bowel movements for earlier in the day.

Avoid coffee, tea, caffeine-containing soft drinks, and alcohol when planning to have sex. Empty your bladder before sex.

You can keep a catheter in during penetration. Men can bring it down along the penis and use a condom; women can tape it out of the way.

Sex in the bathtub or shower is an excellent way of easing into dealing with body fluids.

Some positions (any that put pressure on the lower abdomen) increase pressure on the bladder. Try being on your side, or with the incontinent person on top.

Rubber sheets are more expensive than plastic ones, but they don't make a crinkly sound.

They often contain latex, so should be avoided by people who are allergic to latex. It's always handy to have a couple of towels on hand.

Ostomies

People with ostomies often worry about sounds, smells, and the bag coming off. Any position that puts pressure or movement on the bag area will increase the chance of it coming off. Most people with ostomies say that a sense of humor is essential when having sex. It is a good idea to tell a prospective partner about the ostomy before actually taking your clothes off, but the timing can be tricky and each person needs to figure out what they are comfortable with.

You probably have already figured out which foods produce more gas and which ones go through your system quickly. These vary from person to person. Avoid these foods on days when you are hoping or planning to have sex.

Some people with ostomies have had the rectum removed. In women, the vagina and uterus can then shift backward, causing different sensations during penetration. Muscles that contract around the anus may have been removed or weakened by surgery, which also may change the way an orgasm feels.

People who have had rectal surgery or who could have inflammation in the rectum should avoid anal penetration.

A stoma should *never* be penetrated as part of sex play.

Hypersensitivity

With a number of disabilities hypersensitive areas are not uncommon. Partners should know not to touch you unexpectedly and that sometimes a regular touch will be unwelcome.

People who have hypersensitivity in the genital area may feel like they have to pee when orgasm is coming. Consider the fact that the feeling of having to pee is a common experience related by women who ejaculate. So that feeling may arise from your bladder's being full and your needing to pee, or it may be that you are one of those women who ejaculates and if you let it go, you would not pee but ejaculate. Or it may be that neither is going to happen, it's just a feeling coming from all the genital stimulation you're getting.

Specific Conditions

There are sexuality issues that arise with specific conditions. These are discussed throughout this book, but there are eight conditions for which we have enough information to devote a section to each. We wish we had more information about many other chronic health conditions and disabilities. With publication of this book, we hope to encourage a larger, ongoing discussion of a wide range of specific concerns related to sexuality and disability.

Arthritis

Dealing with pain during sexual activity may involve careful positioning and propping, stopping for a break, or taking a hot bath before sex. Sexual activity increases the output of cortisol from the adrenal glands, which may help alleviate pain.

Swollen painful joints, muscular atrophy, and joint contractures may make masturbation or having sex in certain positions difficult. Creative sexual positioning may reduce pain and pressure on affected joints. Sex toys that are lightweight or easy to hold can help with masturbation. Strap-on vibrators (often called "butterflies") will leave the hands free, but the controls may be tiny and difficult to manipulate.

Pain, fatigue, and medication may decrease one's sex drive, even as genital sensations continue.

Some women with arthritis report that a good position for cunnilingus or penetration is with their legs hanging over the bed and partner kneeling on the floor in front of them.

Cerebral Palsy

The sections in this chapter that address mobility and spasticity cover many of the concerns that people with cerebral palsy (CP) have expressed about sex.

Uncontrollable movements (athetosis) can lead to moments that are either humorous or distressing, depending on how each partner views them.

Activities that involve large movements usually work better than small manipulations.

An athetotic tongue can be great for kissing, oral sex, and stimulation of nipples.

Cystic Fibrosis

Delayed growth and development are common in teens with cystic fibrosis (CF), as a result of nutritional problems. Teens may feel like sexually mature people, but others may view them as still being children because of their appearance.

Coughing is a problem for me even before I get to the sexual stage with someone. Even when I'm dating, I worry about what someone is going to think when I'm coughing up big gobs of mucus. I carry a Ziploc bag or two in my purse, and try to discreetly cough into the bag. I either try to throw a full bag in the garbage or just take it home. I had a boyfriend for a while and it seemed silly to keep hiding it, so I just said, "Look, I cough up mucus, you fart, I think we can each deal with these things." He thought that was pretty funny.

Both men and women with CF report that sex play can lead to increased coughing. It is a good idea to warn partners about this in advance. People with any kind of breathing problems may find that it is uncomfortable to have someone lying on top of them. If you really want to be on the bottom, have your partner use their arms or elbows to support themselves.

Women with CF often have thicker vaginal secretions than other women. Lubricants can be helpful.

Decreased energy can be a big challenge. See tips on energy earlier in this chapter.

Diabetes

Good diabetic control leads to a decrease in the complications that can produce difficulties in getting and maintaining erections.

Retrograde ejaculation, where the semen goes into the bladder instead of coming out the urethra, is common in diabetes. Less common are painful erections, which can be helped by massaging the perineum.

Women with diabetes may be more susceptible to yeast infections because of increased sugar levels in the vagina for the yeast to feed off. These can lead to reduced lubrication, odor, itching, and soreness. Lactobacillus acidophilus capsules inserted into the vagina for a few days after each period can help prevent yeast infections. These are available at most health food stores and should be refrigerated.

About a third of women with diabetes report that orgasms gradually become rarer and less intense. It may be that there is damage to the nerve fibers in the pelvic region, increasing the threshold of nerve signals needed for orgasm. A vibrator may increase likelihood of orgasm, because of the intense stimulation it provides.

Epilepsy

Some people find that sexual arousal or some sexual activities can precipitate a seizure. This can create a situation in which you actively try not to get aroused. It may be that this only happens when other triggers are present, like fatigue or forgetting your medications. If this is the case, then you can work on the other triggers and still let yourself become aroused. Or, depending on what your seizures are like, it may be worth it to you to risk a seizure to have sex.

Many anticonvulsants can interfere with the efficacy of oral contraceptives for women. Alternative forms of birth control should be used, or birth control pills should be combined with other methods. These drugs can also decrease interest in sex and the ability to maintain erections.

Because epilepsy is not an obvious disability, people with epilepsy may keep it a secret. But if there is a chance of a seizure during sexual activity, partners should be told and coached on what to do (and not to do) in the event that one occurs.

Multiple Sclerosis

Many possible symptoms of multiple sclerosis (MS) have been described, and all can affect sexuality, including fatigue, depression, bladder and bowel incontinence, decreased or increased sensation, muscle weakness, spasticity, and tremor, to name just a few. Medications can also have sexual side effects. The good news is that many people with MS have satisfying sex lives.

Planning for sex with MS is more complicated than for some other conditions because it is so unpredictable. Ongoing communication is vital as what feels good changes from day to day or year to year. If you feel more energetic at a certain time of day (the morning perhaps), that's a good time to plan to have sex. A nap afterward will help restore energy.

It may take longer to achieve orgasm, and sometimes it may not be possible. Having the goal of enjoyment rather than orgasm will not decrease the chance of orgasm but may decrease anxiety about sex.

Men may have erectile problems that come and go. This book is full of suggestions of nonpenetrative activities, and the chapter on penetration (chapter 8) talks about possible solutions for erectile difficulties.

Women may have numbness in the genital area, and may need more stimulation to reach orgasm. Some women with MS use a vibrator during sex with a partner.

Tips on incontinence, spasticity, and fatigue can be found in earlier sections of this chapter.

A lack of coordination may make masturbation more of a challenge, though a change to a vibrator with a large head can be helpful, as placement does not have to be exact.

Spinal Cord Injury

More has been written about sex and spinal cord injury (SCI) than any other disability. Much of it is about gender and sexual performance, and how paralysis from SCI challenges traditional gender expectations (that is, the man will be dominant and controlling, the woman giving and attentive). In the midst of all these messages about how we are supposed to be and how now we can't meet these expectations, no one asks what we *want*.

Gender role stereotypes are not written in stone. Many people did not fit these roles before SCI, and some people examine the whole idea and reject it after SCI.

Furthermore, our societal expectations of what real sex is do not have to apply to any of us. Whether or not a man can get an erection or a woman can have an orgasm from clitoral stimulation does not define them as to their sexual potential.

Reduced genital sensation (or no sensation) typically occurs in SCI, depending on the level and severity of the injury. Some men still get erections, others don't. Women may have decreased vaginal lubrication, which can lead to vaginal irritation or even tearing. Bladder infections in both men and women may also make intercourse uncomfortable. Sensation and muscle contraction varies a good deal, so experimentation will help each person figure out their own unique abilities.

Transferring from wheelchair and positioning may require more help than your sexual partner can provide, entailing the help of a third person when you're planning to have sex out of your wheelchair.

As noted in a previous section, catheters and leg bags can be kept on during any sexual activity.

Many people notice areas of increased sensitivity just about the line where they lose sensation. Having this area stroked, licked, or tickled can be very sexually pleasurable. After SCI, people often discover how much sexual pleasure they can get from their lips, earlobes, nipples, armpits, inner elbows, and neck.

Skin ulcers are another concern. Prolonged pressure on a part of the body where there is no sensation can cut off the blood flow to the skin, leading to ulcers, as can friction. Partners need to be aware of this and change positions frequently.

Women may continue to have orgasms regardless of level or degree of paralysis. These orgasms may be similar to those before injury or may be felt in places other than the genitals, either all over the body or in a specific place like the breasts or lips. Some women find that cervical stimulation (with penetration by a sex toy or penis) can induce an orgasm even in the absence of genital sensation.

Be on guard for autonomic dysreflexia (AD), which can lead to a life-threatening disruption of the autonomic nervous system marked by increased spasms and chills. This is discussed in chapter 12.

Stroke

One of the big sexual fears of people who have had a stroke is that sex will bring on another one. This is unlikely, and if another stroke in going to happen, it will do so with or without sex.

Language problems (both speaking and understanding) after a stroke can interfere with sexual communication, and nonverbal signals may need to be developed.

If balance, strength, or coordination are poor, sexual activities that require little exertion can be tried. These would include anything where the body is supported.

Decreased interest in sex can happen after a stroke, and cues of sexual arousal might be missed. Being willing to have sex, even if you aren't sure you are aroused, is one way to get around this. Erection issues include not being able to maintain an erection and taking more or less time to ejaculate. An erection that comes and goes is not a barrier to great sex when you are having nonpenetrative sex.

7

Oral Sex

A great story is told about Connie Panzarino, an American disability activist, who marched one year in a gay pride parade with a big sign proclaiming "TRACHED LESBIANS CAN EAT PUSSY FOR HOURS."

Oral sex is considered by many to be the most physically intimate sex act possible. Partners can see, smell, and taste each other's genitals. The experience can be intense and gratifying, yet it may make some people feel vulnerable and exposed. As with everything else, feeling comfortable with what you are doing is an important starting place. For some people it can take a long time to enjoy receiving and giving oral sex.

I have a hard time with relationships because I don't really understand all these wild emotions people seem to have. But I do like having sex. Sometimes regular sex is overwhelming. There is just too much to take in all at once. My autism makes this a problem. Oral sex is great because there it's just one area to focus on. I close my eyes and just feel and smell and explore every little nook and cranny. My last lover said that she never felt like she had to hurry to come because she knew I loved doing it and liked having lots of time.

In many ways oral sex is ideally suited for people with disabilities. It may get around issues of spasticity, low energy, problems with erections, positioning needs, lubrication, and anything that makes penetration difficult or uncomfortable. And, as Panzarino's sign points out, some of us are particularly gifted at doing things with our mouths for hours without having to come up for air!

At the same time, our genitals are often the site of a lot of negativity, ranging from unpleasant messages to abuse. Some of us were told that our genitals were only for reproduction. Or others assumed that we could never have children and therefore our genitals should be ignored entirely (except to keep them clean). We have been told they are dirty, ugly, or smelly. Girls have been given the message that we should only notice our genitals when taking care of our periods.

In addition to this, many of us have had experiences with caregivers and professionals touching and looking at our genitals on a regular basis in connection to bladder and bowel routines. All this may make this part of the body one that makes us feel awkward and anxious.

Because of the physical structure of women's genitals, they are mostly hidden from view. Many women (and their partners) will have sex without ever really looking at their own genitals. While most men have better access to their genitals, it is still informative and exciting for them to get feedback about the area. Communicating about the look, feel, smell, or taste of someone's genitals may be difficult at first, but they are likely to love hearing it.

Giving and receiving oral sex can be a positive step toward changing our relationship with this part of our body. Specific techniques aside, just the act of paying close and loving attention to your partner's genitals can be intensely exciting for both partners.

Another exciting thing about oral sex it that it is a sensation that is impossible to replicate on one's own. The feel of a finger is much different than that of a flexible, warm, wet tongue.

> *I am thirty-nine years old and married. My wife and I have a satisfactory sex life. I now have a penile prosthesis, which I had surgically implanted when I was about thirty-two. We have genital sex often, and I enjoy giving her oral sex. When I engage in cunnilingus with my wife, she just about always reaches orgasm. My face becomes moist with her vaginal secretions, and she becomes wet all over her entire pubis and inside the cleft of her buttock. This wetness is the visible sign of her pleasure. When it is my own turn to be pleasured, I try to imagine myself and my wife covered in the wetness of my own sperm. Since I do not have sensation in my penis, and I cannot ejaculate sperm, the best I can do is to conjure up some mental image, and thus we rely on fantasy as part of our sexual repertoire in order to add to the arousal.*

Before we dive into this chapter we want to make a note about the language we use here. For ease in description we refer to the "giver" and the "receiver." Sometimes people who haven't enjoyed oral sex before think of it as an activity that involves one person doing a job (the giver) and the other person enjoying themselves (the receiver). In fact most people who give oral sex a try end up loving both sides of it.

Common Concerns

Appearance

It is the rare person who was raised to feel proud about their gorgeous genitalia. The best way to begin dealing with negative images is to get a chance to take a good look for yourself. See chapter 3 for tips on this. Whether you get the chance to see what you look like, or feel what you look like, try to discover at least one thing about your genitals that you like.

In addition to understanding your own body and how you feel about it, be respectful of how your partner is feeling about him or herself. With all the shame and guilt they may feel about their genitals, they may not be comfortable with the idea of receiving oral sex. If your partner feels this way, don't take it as an insult or an indication that you are being rejected. Respect their need to go at their own pace, while you provide support and positive feedback about their desirability.

Smell and Taste

All the messages we've taken in about our genitals set us up for finding things wrong with what's "down there." Two of the most common concerns people have is smell and taste. It seems as if men in particular have a lot of preconceived ideas of what women's genitals smell like. This is not usually based on actual experience, and most men find that once they try it they like it far more than they expected.

> I was married for a while and my husband would never go down on me 'cause he said it smelled. I believed him because I knew that it was a gross part of my body. A while ago I started sleeping with someone who really wanted to go down on me. I wouldn't let him because I didn't want him to be grossed out. But one night when we smoked some dope I let him and he loved how I taste. He said it was tangy, not gross at all. And I felt like I was having sex for the first time, it was so great and not like anything I had ever felt.

There are sweat glands in the genital area that, over the course of the day, can generate a lot of perspiration. A different odor can result, particularly if you wear clothes that are tight or not very breathable, and if you spend most of the day in a seated position. You can do a couple of things about this, but again we want to propose that much of the hesitation about oral sex is based on people's expectations rather than experience. The first thing you can try to do is time a bath or shower just before you're going to have sex (particularly if it's after a long, sweaty day). Ideally, make the cleaning up part of the sex play. Both the bathtub and the shower are great places for sex, and even if you're not doing it with your partner, cleaning yourself can be a kind of solo foreplay, getting yourself geared up for the excitement to come.

You should also be aware that an unpleasant smell may be the result of an infection; if it persists it may be worth checking out with your doctor.

If you use lubricant during sex play be aware that some kinds taste sweet, while others have a bitter taste. If your partner complains about your taste, it could be the lube.

Finally, we should point out that a lot of sex educators recommend using condoms and dental dams for oral sex, and these barriers also block genital taste and smell.

Because people have a lot of expectations about going down on someone, much of it negative, we recommend taking the pressure off oral sex by leaving it for later on in sex play. Don't make it the first thing you do after kissing, because you both may still be a little hesitant and feel awkward. If you wait until you're both fully turned on, with your inhibitions down a bit, a lot of the negative expectations will be gone. Another good reason to take some time before going down is that some people say that the more excited a woman is, the sweeter her natural lubrication is.

Incontinence

Bowel and bladder incontinence are a huge concern for many people. See chapter 6 for a longer discussion on this topic, as well as tips on ways of dealing with it. For some people incontinence is a bigger issue with oral sex because someone is right there, and there's less of a chance that your partner won't notice if your body releases some urine or feces as a response to being turned on or excited. The best thing to do is to avoid having a full bladder or rectum when you are going to be receiving oral sex. This may mean catheterizing just before sex, and avoiding alcohol or caffeine if you're thinking about having sex in the next few hours. They are both diuretics, so your bladder will fill up more quickly.

The Gag Reflex

Almost all of us have a gag reflex. It occurs in a spot in the throat that makes us gag or want to throw up when it is touched. The gag reflex is more an issue with *fellatio* (going down on a man) than *cunnilingus* (going down on a woman). The size of the mouth cavity is almost always smaller than the size of the penis. So when many of us try to take someone's entire penis in our mouths we encounter the gag reflex. Fellatio doesn't have to include taking his cock all the way in your mouth. Still, this technique, called "deep throating," is one that a lot of people can learn, and several books and websites (noted in the resources chapter) offer tips on mastering it. But not everyone can learn to get past their gag reflex, nor is deep throating the be-all and end-all of oral sex.

Cunnilingus

One of the most exciting aspects of sex is anticipation. Wondering what's going to happen next, becoming aware of what one hopes will come next, and being surprised are all part of this. Going down on a woman is as much about having a sense of adventure and exploration as it is knowing the right thing to do, and when.

> *I enjoy sex and foreplay probably as much as anyone else does. My husband and I both enjoy giving and receiving oral sex, and genital intercourse. Orgasm is certainly important to me—can't imagine sex without it. I'm pretty lucky. I'm multiply orgasmic and have an orgasm every time my husband pleasures me. I need direct clitoral stimulation to climax, so traditional intercourse is pleasant but generally doesn't make me come, unless I'm also using a vibrator. Receiving oral is my favorite and always gets the job done.*

Getting the Lay of the Land

If you are a bit unsure about what everything is "down there," now might be a good time to go back to chapter 3 and check out the picture of female genitals. Their appearance varies from one woman to the next, so take your time with your partner and really check her out. You can use your lips, tongue, mouth, and other parts of your face and head to explore the whole area. If both of you are comfortable with it, start with the lights on so that you can really see what's going on and where you are.

While most people prefer external stimulation, you don't have to limit your explorations to what is immediately accessible to you. You can use your tongue to explore not only the varied folds of skin but also what's immediately inside your partner's vagina. Many people enjoy penetration while receiving oral sex, and fingers or toys are perfect for just this purpose. Ask your partner whether this is something she's comfortable with.

As you're exploring don't forget to keep other kinds of communication open. If you happen to be having a grand time with your discoveries, be sure to let your partner know (a moan is often as good as a verbal compliment for feedback). It's also great to hear from the receiver what feels good and what doesn't. You can experiment with different kinds of communication. Some people will be comfortable talking, explicitly saying what works and doesn't for them. But breathing, moaning, using your hands to guide your partner's head—all are equally useful ways to communicate what you want, or what you want to try.

I love it when I can watch my boyfriend go down on me. Sometimes he'll look up at me, or just open his eyes and have this look of being delirious with excitement, and it turns me on even more. I think I'd like it if he made a little more noise, but as long as I can see his face and he's busy working away, I'm satisfied with it.

As we discussed in chapter 3, for most women the clitoris is the site of the greatest sensitivity. If your partner enjoys clitoral stimulation, it would be good to find out what kind of stimulation she likes the best. Some women enjoy direct stimulation over the clitoris; others prefer it to the side (sometimes even a particular side). Some like gentle stimulation, while others need and love strong pressure.

If neither of you has stated a preference, why not just experiment with different kinds of stimulation? You can use your tongue to gently brush or nudge the clitoris, you can slowly lick her clitoris with the flat part of your tongue, or lick only the sides of the clitoris. You can put her clitoris in your mouth and gently (or not so gently) suck. Play with different tongue strokes. One suggestion is to use your tongue to spell out the alphabet, which allows for a wide variety of tonguing directions, leading to all kinds of delightful discoveries. You can start by running your tongue from the bottom of the vulva right up to her clitoris. Everybody is different, but most women have folds of skin that will love to be licked or sucked. Some people will enjoy gentle tugging too.

You will recall that the clitoris is covered by the clitoral hood. Some women love to have their clitoris more directly stimulated, while others find it uncomfortable or even painful. If you've got a free hand, you can use it to gently pull up on the skin just above the clitoris. Doing this will pull back the clitoral hood and will expose the clitoris more than it normally would be exposed. Then lick gently, paying attention to your partner's response. Another sensitive area for some women is right around the urethra.

You don't have to ignore other parts of your partner's body. Whatever you have access to, you can stimulate during oral sex. You can reach up and stroke her breasts or belly. You may want to slip a finger in her vagina, or her anus, or both. Many women also like having the area around their vulva and pubic bone touched and massaged during oral sex.

Gently separate her outer lips with your tongue, or use your fingers if that's easier. You'll want to locate her clitoris, but you don't have to pounce on it.

Try using your face and head to nuzzle in between her legs. You can use your nose as a sex toy, rubbing it against her clitoris or flooding the area with moist, warm air.

Probably because of my meds I find that my mouth gets really dry when I'm giving my girlfriend head. The simple solution we came up with was to have a squirt bottle of water by the bed at all times. I sometimes have to take a breather, but if the water is cold I can also use it to my advantage when I go back down.

Positioning

For everyone, finding the right position for cunnilingus takes imagination and creativity. A sense of humor also helps. There isn't one position that everyone likes, and the position must suit both partners. The most traditional position for cunnilingus is with the receiver on her back with the giver lying between her legs. A pillow under her butt might bring her vulva into a position that will be more comfortable for the giver's neck. Sitting in a chair, or the edge of a bed or couch, can also work well if the giver can comfortably kneel. Or the giver can lie on their back with a pillow under their head while the receiver is on her knees over the giver's face. The person on top can be supported by the wall or headboard, or by hardware such as a wall-mounted grab bar or a bar suspended from the ceiling.

The right position at one moment is not always the right position forever. Some women love to receive oral sex in a position where they are upright or on top, but can't have an orgasm unless their body is more supported, so they will want to shift positions at some point. Also, either person may find a limb going numb, neck getting sore, or a muscle cramping somewhere. "I need to change positions" doesn't mean "I want to stop."

The tips on positions in chapter 8 may apply as well here as they do for penetration.

Tips and Technique

As you explore you'll find different things that your partner loves. Don't feel you have to stick to the same motion, but do try to get a sense of whether your partner wants a change. Repeated rhythmic tongue strokes are what get many women over the top, so you don't want to change what you are doing too frequently. Be aware of your partner's rising and falling pleasure. Try to tune into her body movements, breathing, or what she might be saying, to learn whether she wants faster or slower, more or less.

It isn't your responsibility alone, however, to know what great oral sex is and what will turn your partner on. She needs to let you know what works and what doesn't.

Someone once said that vulvas are like snowflakes: No two are exactly alike. Take the time to appreciate what's before you, and offer some signs of appreciation. Tell her what you like about her vulva, her clit, what looks good or feels good. Moans of wild excitement will do just as well as a hundred words.

Your partner may feel turned on by watching you or by eye contact. She may enjoy it if you look at her, as long as you don't stop what you are doing. If it's difficult for you to have direct eye contact in a certain position, mirrors (either a small hand-held one or one mounted on the wall or on a floor stand) can allow you both to see what you want without causing pain to your necks or backs.

Some people wonder when to stop. It isn't always clear when a woman has had an orgasm or when she is physically spent and wants to change to something else. Some women like you to stop after her orgasm, others like you to keep going. She might want you to continue the same way, especially if she is hoping for another orgasm, or she might want you to slow down or just press your tongue on her clit. You can't guess what she wants, so she needs to let you know with words or signals, like pressing on your head gently.

Fellatio

As with cunnilingus, when it comes to sucking cock, anticipation is key, and working slowly toward the penis is a good idea. When you get there, take a look at the penis in front of you. You may never have had a chance to do this before, or it might be old hat to you, but either way keep in mind that like every vulva, every cock is different. Take the time to feel around every fold of skin, nook, and cranny with your fingers and your tongue. This can be exciting for both partners.

Getting the Lay of the Land

One of the biggest differences in penises is whether they are circumcised or not. In uncircumcised penises, the head of the penis is hidden under the foreskin when the penis is not erect. An uncircumcised penis has more skin to move around and play with, and it's less likely that an enthusiastic tug or pull will hurt. The head of an uncircumcised penis is more sensitive to touch. By contrast, a benefit of a circumcised penis is that it's all right out there, whether or not it's erect, and you get easier access to all its parts.

Having reviewed the anatomy in chapter 3 (do this now, not while you are having sex!), you will want to learn your partner's particular topography. Find out where he is the most sensitive, how and where he likes to be touched.

The area under the head of the penis where the head meets the shaft (called the *frenulum*) is often the most sensitive spot. It has the greatest concentration of nerve endings, while the shaft of the penis has fewer nerve endings and less sensation. Although some men enjoy both the look and feel of vigorous friction on the shaft, most will want some kind of stimulation of the rest of the penis to get off. The *testicles* (balls) can be very sensitive to touch and pressure and can be stimulated orally.

Once you've got an idea of all the parts you're working with, you can start exploring. Start wherever is most comfortable for you and work your way either up or down the penis, the head, shaft, and balls, slowly using your mouth, tongue, lips, to touch every part of him. As you move slowly pay attention to his reactions. Even if he doesn't give you verbal feedback, you'll get a good idea from his body responses what is turning him on.

Fellatio also doesn't have to be just about the genitals. If you have access to other parts of his body, touching, stroking, lightly running nails along the skin or playing with his nipples can add extra stimulation and expand the experience of oral sex for both of you.

Positioning

My favorite position is with the guy sitting on my chest, with me sucking his cock, sucking his balls, eating his ass, and ending by him jerking off.

One thing that works for us is when I lie at the end of the bed, my stomach on the bed and my waist and legs off the bed. She then

*sits on the floor with her back to the bed and sort of lies under me
and can play with me that way.*

The position you choose should be comfortable for both the giver
and the receiver. You'll get the most access to all parts of his penis if you
are between his legs. It may be most comfortable for him to be on his
back in bed with you lying or kneeling between his legs. It might be better for you to be on top of him. He can sit on the edge of the bed or a
chair, or be in one of many positions on a couch. If you use a wheelchair
it may be possible for you to give oral sex in your wheelchair with your
partner lying on a bed or table that's the right height for you. A wheelchair can also be a perfect place to be on the receiving end. As always,
pillows can be helpfully placed under someone's butt or under the knees,
to either raise someone up or make kneeling or sitting more comfortable.

Tips and Technique

Don't rely on one motion only, or focus on one part of the penis only.
Mix it up, both in terms of what you're stimulating and the pacing of the
stimulation.

Sometimes people think that fellatio means putting a cock in your
mouth and moving your head up and down, with some occasional sucking action. It can be this, but it can also be much, much more. Don't forget to use your tongue. Play with different movements, lick clockwise for
a bit, and then counterclockwise. You can rub his penis along the sides
of your teeth in the pouch that your cheek makes. There is much to be
said for subtlety. Try using your tongue to gently flick the head of the
penis, starting slow and ending up with some fast and furious flicking. If
you flutter your tongue up and down on the underside of his penis while
it's in your mouth, you may be amazed by the reaction.

When you take his cock in your mouth, take it in slowly, using your
tongue as a guide. If you can, wrap a hand around the shaft while his
cock is sliding into your mouth. You can move your head around his
cock, either in circles or up and down. You can let his cock slip all the
way out of your mouth and back in, or keep it in your mouth for longer
without taking it out.

Once the receiver is comfortable and excited, you can start playing more with his balls. Testicles are very sensitive to both pleasure and pain, and react badly to any threat. So go slowly with them. Try alternating licking and sucking to see if either or both are pleasurable for him. You can take both balls into your mouth at the same time or one at a time. Many men like the feeling of having their balls held or cupped.

> *My boyfriend goes crazy when someone holds his balls while giving him head. I can't always do this so I have him sitting down and before I start to suck I take a small towel, get it wet with warm water, and then wrap it around his balls. Sometimes I just use the towel without the water. I can usually manage to squeeze the towel a bit and nudge it with my mouth and face. I don't know what it does for him, but I know he likes it!*

Another technique is to make a ring shape with your hand at the top of the scrotum, holding just the skin. Very slowly and gently pull down away from his belly, while still playing with the rest of his penis. It is safe to pull harder if he wants, providing you are not putting pressure on the testicles, but just pulling on the skin.

The perineum, the area behind the balls and between the scrotum and the anus, is often quite sensitive. You can lick this area or gently massage it. Some men don't like this, but you won't know if you don't try. Try grabbing his penis near the base and pull up (toward his belly), exposing his balls, then lick from the perineum all the way up the shaft to the head of his dick.

> *I once was giving this guy head and he had his legs pulled back showing his rear entrance and asked me to stick my hand up as far as possible. I wasn't into that but used the dildo and when he came it was a different rush, inserting the dildo as far as possible and feeling him cum down my throat. I would definitely do that again!*

Some men really like anal stimulation but are afraid to ask for it. Inserting one or more fingers in his ass while focusing your mouth on his cock can be heaven for many men. Some men describe the feeling of having their penis stimulated while being penetrated as having "two cocks," one inside and one outside.

Spit or Swallow?

For some people this is a big issue. Some men feel it is a form of ultimate acceptance if their partner swallows their cum. Other men don't care one way or another. If you are using a condom, then you will not be confronted with the issue of what to do if and when your partner ejaculates. Many people do not want to swallow semen, and some are uncomfortable having a man ejaculate in their mouth. This is an issue of personal choice. You can always spit it out (have some tissues ready). Once you are familiar with a partner you may be able to anticipate ejaculation by a few clues. The noises he makes and body movements are good indicators. For a lot of men another sign is that the head of the cock will swell just prior to ejaculating. Often a small amount of semen will come out just before ejaculation. This is referred to as pre-cum.

> The way I deal with guys who want me to swallow is simple. I tell them I'll swallow if they will. I figure hey, if I'm willing to taste and swallow their cum, they should be too, so before I swallow they have to take some also. If they refuse, then so do I. It just seems fair, and some of my partners have really got off on it.

Mutual Oral Sex (the 69 Position)

The *"69 position"* allows for both partners to stimulate each other's genitals at the same time. It can be a fun variation on oral sex. One main obstacle is finding a position that will be comfortable for both of you. A second typical complaint about this activity is that one partner usually slows down as a result of wanting to focus on the pleasure they are receiving. There are no great tried-and-true positions that will work for everyone, and this position seems to get the most attention in porn, rather than in real people's sex lives. That said, getting creative and trying to satisfy both partners' needs at the same time can be a fun project for an evening, or afternoon, or weekend.

Analingus

Oral/anal contact is called *analingus,* also referred to as *rimming*. Many people find it highly pleasurable. It is also considered to be quite risky in terms of transmitting infections. If you want to try this we recommend you use a barrier between your mouth and your partner's anus. See chapter 12 on safer sex and sexual health for a longer discussion of this. Before you skip over this section completely, remember that people who have little or no genital sensation may still have plenty of feeling in and around the anus, so exploring this kind of play can open up a lot of new possibilities for pleasure.

First, the area should completely clean. If you know you want to explore this part of your partner's body, try to arrange that they bathe or shower just before. The receiver should ensure that the area around their asshole is clean, and if possible try to clean the area immediately inside the anus just by inserting a wet finger in their rectum a bit and then washing it off well.

The ideal position is obviously one that exposes the ass as much as possible. The receiver may be in a chair, or on the edge of the bed, or on their back. Their legs can be the air or over the giver's shoulders. The giver could be on their back with the receiver over them. The receiver can be on their belly over a pile of pillows.

As we will be discussing in chapter 8, anal contact does not have to mean penetration. Oral/anal contact may not involve actually putting your tongue in someone's anus, especially because there are many nerve endings on the skin around the anus. You can begin very gently and slowly, even with just your breath. You can also use your nose to lightly brush up against the anus. Anal/oral contact is usually less of a sucking action and more of a caress. Let your tongue pass up and down along the anus, or twirl your tongue in circles starting farther away from the anus and moving slowly closer to the ridgey area right around the anus.

You may want to insert a finger or toy into your partner's anus while licking or sucking other parts of their genitals.

Using Toys

While oral sex is usually about the mouth, there's nothing that says you can't add other elements to oral play. Some people like to use a vibrator during oral sex. Anything from a large plug-in massager to the tiny vibrators that fit on your fingers can add pizzazz to oral sex. The vibrator can be guided by either partner. It can be placed on any part of the penis or vulva that isn't being stimulated with the mouth, and moved around on the inner thighs, perineum, ass, belly, chest, or nipples, wherever it feels good. Dildos can be used for vaginal penetration, and butt plugs can be used anally during oral sex. Chapter 9 covers many aspects of sex toy use.

Kissing

You might not think of kissing in connection with oral sex, but it *is* sex and it's done with mouths, so we thought this would be a good place to mention it. Kissing is a great sexual act. You can get totally turned on without ever taking off your clothes, you can go on and on for a long time. Need we say that there are about a million different ways to kiss? And even better, there has never been a documented case of HIV being spread by kissing.

Positioning

Any position where two mouths are in close proximity will work. You don't want to get into a position where someone's nose is blocked. Kissing can be done standing, sitting, reclining, or lying down. When lying side by side, each person has to figure out a comfortable position for the arm on the bottom. If one person is going to lie on top of the other, the person on top needs to be aware of how much pressure they are putting on the other person. This is particularly important if the person on the bottom has decreased or absent sensation and would not be able to tell if their leg is being crushed. Kissing in a wheelchair also requires some maneuvering. If both people are in chairs, getting close enough can be a problem, so your best bet is with the chairs next to each other but facing in opposite directions, a kind of "wheelchair 69." If one person isn't in a chair, then they can lean over for a short period of time. This position has implications of dominance, which may be uncomfortable for some, and a major turn-on for others. Another possibility is for one person to sit on the lap of the other. This position requires that the person on the bottom have strong bones. If one partner is much taller than the other, a good position can be with the shorter person sitting on a counter while the taller one stands.

> My girlfriend doesn't use a wheelchair but she figured out how we can kiss for a quite a while without either one of us feeling uncomfortable. One way is she gets on her knees so she's at the right height as me. This isn't something she can do for long, but it does feel more equal between us…also I can reach parts of her upper body with my lips that I can't when we're kissing and she's leaning over me in my wheelchair. Another way is that she'll sit on a chair and have me wheel up in front of her so she can straddle my chair. I feel more at ease knowing she's comfortable.

Technique

Perhaps more than any other sexual activity, kissing is a kind of sex that simply can't be rushed. In the throes of passion kissing may get rough and aggressive, but when first kissing someone your best bet is gentle exploration and subtle technique. Kissing can involve just the lips: pressed to each other gently or firmly, rubbed against each other, nibbled with or on. A kiss not only feels good for the receiver, but as the kisser you can sense your partner's body and response in a different way. When you kiss someone's lips, face, wherever on their body you like and they like, notice what their skin feels like under your lips. Kissing can also involve the tongue. This is often called *French kissing*. This can be done either with the couple's lips pressed together or with them in more casual contact. The more casual contact works well for people who can only breathe through their mouths, for they can keep breathing while kissing. The tongues can touch and tease each other, or a tongue can be run over the lips or gums of the other person. You can also get your teeth involved, mixing up soft kisses and touches of tongues with gentle (and possibly not so gentle) nibbles and bites.

Some people like to have their eyes open while kissing, to see their partner's face. Others prefer to have their eyes closed, or find it overwhelming to be looked at during kissing.

We know one sex educator who tells people who want to practice kissing without a partner to use marshmallows, pudding, and other small candy. Take some in your mouth and try to roll it around your mouth and play with it without chewing or dissolving it at first. Partly this can be a game of keeping the food in your mouth and not swallowing it. But it can also be a way of experimenting with the many enticing things your lips, tongue, teeth, and mouth can do.

8

Penetration and Positioning

Sex is often defined as a man putting his penis in his partner's vagina. Some people who are very sexually active may think that they have never had "real" sex because they haven't engaged in penis-in-vagina penetration.

True, penetration can be an enjoyable part of sex, but we can have real sex without ever penetrating someone or being penetrated. Penetration does not have to involve a penis. We can use our fingers, hands, an assortment of perfectly safe vegetables, and many kinds of sex toys for penetration.

People like penetration for all sorts of reasons. Many experience it as an intense form of physical intimacy, allowing for a lot of body-to-body contact. Penetration has many psychological implications as well. Allowing someone to penetrate us, trusting them enough to literally open our bodies up to them, can be a powerful form of sharing. Some heterosexual men are opening themselves up to the experience of being penetrated by their female partners and discovering the pleasure and intimacy it creates.

Many people simply like the way penetration feels. Even if you have little or no external genital sensation, you may enjoy, and get off from, being penetrated. While it is in no way an essential part of sex, if you're interested in it there is no reason not to experiment— even if you have had doctors tell you "It won't work" or "You won't feel anything."

Vaginal Penetration

Some women orgasm easily with penetration by fingers, a whole hand, a penis, or a sex toy. Most women do not have orgasms from penetration alone, but when combined with cli-

BEND OVER, BOYFRIEND

A few years ago, several people associated with the sex store Good Vibrations were inspired to create an educational video geared to heterosexual couples who wanted to explore male anal play. The inspiration came from the large number of people who were going to sex stores and asking about the how's and why's of women penetrating men anally. The result is an excellent video, called Bend Over Boyfriend (known as BOB, for short), that combines education with sex. BOB offers instruction and explicit demonstration of technique, role-playing and fantasy, and how to communicate with your partner, plus tips on how to shop for toys for play. It is hosted by sex educators Carol Queen and Robert Morgan, and has become a huge bestseller, so much so that BOB 2 was produced not long after the first tape came out. Most of the stores listed in the Sexuality: Products section of chapter 14 have this video for sale, and it is also available through Fatale Media (www.fatalemedia.com), the company that produced the first volume.

toral and other kinds of stimulation, they may have orgasms while being penetrated. During orgasm the muscles circling the vagina contract, and these contractions may be felt more strongly if there is something in the vagina. There are many possible positions for vaginal penetration, and we will explore some of them below.

Despite the widely held belief that first penetration is painful, it isn't always so, especially if the woman is aroused and well lubricated. Taking things slowly at first also helps. Some women have a painful reaction to penetration, called *vaginismus*. With vaginismus the muscles in the vagina spasm, making penetration difficult (or impossible) and very painful. Vaginismus can be treated effectively in several ways that don't involve medication, so if penetration is painful you may want to find a registered sex therapist to talk to about this. See the Sexuality: Health and Safer Sex section of chapter 14.

We highly recommend using a lubricant for all kinds of vaginal penetration. Fingers, hands, and toys do not lubricate themselves, but even if you are having intercourse (penetration by a penis) lubrication makes everything more wet, more comfortable, and often more fun.

Fingers

While not everyone will be able to use their fingers and hands to penetrate a partner, if you can, it's a great way to start exploring penetration. One of the nice things about using fingers is that you get to feel more of what's going on inside your partner. Penises are not as sensitive as fingers and hands (and of course dildos are not sensitive at all), and while you can always gauge your partners' reaction by how they respond, having the opportunity to really "get in there" can be useful and exciting.

If you are going to penetrate your partner with your fingers, you need to start by removing any and all jewelry, make sure your nails are short and clean, and check to see if you have any cuts on your fingers or hands. One concern is that if you penetrate someone while wearing a ring, or if you have very long or jagged nails, you could cut your partner. A second concern is that if you have open cuts on your hands you are at risk for getting a sexually transmitted infection (STI) (see chapter 12 for more safer sex tips). The easiest way to deal with both these concerns is to use latex or nonlatex rubber gloves for penetration. In chapter 12 we list the options for people with latex and other allergies. Gloves make everything smooth, they don't reduce sensation that much, and they also act as a barrier to STIs.

You can use your fingers however your partner likes. There is a huge variation in the way people like to be penetrated by fingers (also called *finger fucking*). Few people like to be poked and prodded, and it's always good to start off gently, and not to forget what's going on outside the vagina. Pay attention to the clitoris and vulva as you move inside your partner. It is perfectly safe to insert several fingers, and even a whole hand, in the vagina, but you need to let your partner be your guide. If you curve your fingers a bit (bending them toward your partner's belly button), you can stimulate her G-spot through finger penetration (which she may like, or may not like, or may not even notice).

Vaginal Fisting

This kind of penetration involves having your entire hand (which curls into the shape of a fist) in your partner's vagina. People on both the giving and the receiving end describe *fisting* as an extremely intense experience. It requires a lot of communication and trust between partners. Despite its name, fisting is not a violent activity, and, if done safely, it is not a dangerous form of sex play. For those of you who find it hard to believe that a whole fist could get in a vagina, keep in mind that newborns are much larger than fists.

Entire books are devoted to fisting, and if you want to experiment with this kind of play we suggest you check out the Sexuality: General Resources section of chapter 14.

Meanwhile, here are some key points to safe vaginal fisting:

- Always use latex or nonlatex gloves.
- Fisting is something that requires a slow buildup, much patience, and lots of lubricant.
- The person doing the fisting needs to be able to keep a steady and consistent movement of the hand that will be going into the vagina. They need another hand free to add lube at regular intervals and to provide clitoral stimulation, if desired. If the person doing the fisting only has one hand available, the person receiving can stimulate herself and can also provide the lubricant.
- Start by inserting one finger at a time. Your palm should be facing your

partner's belly. Don't rush this. Go slow and tease until you have four fingers sliding comfortably in and out of your partner's vagina. Remember to add lube to both your gloved hand and your partner while you are playing.

- While you are working up to four fingers your partner can experiment with "bearing down" on her vaginal muscles, which will open her up a bit more and draw your fingers deeper into her. She may also want to try to synchronize her breathing with your motions.
- It is a good idea to use a variety of movements with your hand, moving in and out, including some twisting motions.
- To get your entire hand in your partner's vagina you need to tuck your thumb across your palm and squeeze your fingers together (you're trying to make your hand as narrow as possible). Some fisters refer to this hand position as the "duck" because you are making your hand look a little like a duck's bill.
- Knuckles are the point of greatest resistance. As always, let your partner guide you here, and wait until she's ready for the final push.
- Once your hand is completely inside her, curl your fingers up to make a fist.

Dildos

Dildos provide all the same possibilities and feelings as penetration with a penis, with the obvious advantage of being able to pick whatever size, shape, and color you like. Your partner might manipulate the dildo with their hands, or they may want to wear a strap-on harness that will allow them "no hands" penetration.

> My girlfriend has CP and isn't able to spread her legs easily or for very long. I have MD and am not able to hold myself on my knees for very long so I can't do it the doggie-style like other guys can. How we get around it is by using a dildo—and my girlfriend loves it when we use her dildo. She is able to stay on her knees and I get in behind her and play with her clit until she is really wet. Then we use the dildo. She says it feels like a penis...I like to think it's mine

inside of her. I can slide the dildo in and out and rub her clit at the same time. She says she comes really hard and fast when I use the dildo and stimulate her inner lips and clit.

For a more detailed discussion of dildos see chapter 9.

Penises

As we've suggested, penis-in-vagina intercourse is usually viewed as the only "real" kind of sex. Because of this incorrect belief, we've spent a lot of time discussing the many other things you can do sexually, activities that don't get talked about as much. But we don't want to put down this kind of sex either. Penetrating your partner with your penis (or being on the receiving end of it) is a very intimate experience, as it allows for a lot of physical contact and touch and thus can feel absolutely wonderful. People who haven't tried penetrative sex sometimes wonder how a penis gets into a vagina. Most of the time either the man or the woman guides it in with their hand. Many people think that to experience this they need to be able to get full erections at a moment's notice. This isn't true.

Sometimes I'll just put my penis inside her even though I don't have a hard-on. It's not like it feels the same but it lets us get very close and we can just rock back and forth and sometimes that will get me turned on enough that I get a hard-on. Even if that doesn't happen, it feels good.

One of the oldest techniques for penetration without an erection is called *stuffing*. With stuffing a man can tuck his penis into his partner's vagina without an erection. By moving her hips and using her PC muscle the woman can create a sort of pulling and sucking experience inside her vagina. At the same time, the man's body moving against the woman can provide clitoral stimulation. This technique is easiest with the man on top and his partner's legs drawn up to her chest.

Other options for penile-vaginal intercourse with a man who isn't getting erections involve medications, pumps, or injections. If you are interested in exploring these options, you can start by asking your reg-

ular doctor (if you think they will be a safe person to ask) for information and, possibly, a referral to a urologist. If you've tried stuffing but
want to further explore vaginal penetration without surgery or drugs,
try playing with harnesses and dildos. There are two kinds of strap-on
toys for men to wear. One kind is a hollow dildo that fits over your
penis and straps around your waist. The second, which we prefer, is a
harness that leaves your penis exposed and places the dildo just slightly
above your penis. The benefit of this kind of harness is that your genitals are still exposed and if you have sensation they can be stimulated
(either by you or your partner). Chapter 9 offers more details about
these toys.

Penetration follows no technical rules. Start with a sense of what
turns you on and how you like to be stimulated—where would you like
to go from there? The most important thing to remember is that penetration, while it might be the focus of the action, doesn't have to be the
sole thing happening. Stimulating other parts of your own and your partner's body while having intercourse will only add to the enjoyment.
Below we suggest a number of positions.

Anal Sex

Many people already think of the ass as a sexy part of the body, but that
usually is restricted to checking each other out, maybe a little bit of rubbing, fondling, or a slap here and there between lovers. There is an old
and deep taboo against anal sex. But the ass—the anus, the anal canal,
and the rectum—can be a source of deep pleasure. People lacking sensation around the penis/scrotum or vulva area can often experience
strong sensation around the anus.

Anal sex doesn't necessarily mean penetration. For the vast majority
of people who try it, anal sex doesn't involve anything more than external stimulation and possibly finger penetration. In chapter 7 we offer
specific information about oral/anal contact. If you are interested in more
information, the Sexuality: General Resources section of chapter 14 cites
three excellent books devoted to anal play: *Anal Pleasure and Health*

by Jack Morin, *The Ultimate Guide to Anal Sex for Women* by Tristan Taormino, and *The Ultimate Guide to Anal Sex for Men* by Bill Brent.

Start by getting to know your anus. The opening of the anus contains the highest concentration of nerve endings. The anus responds to feelings of fullness or pressure, and many people like the feeling of fingers, dildos, and penises in their anus. When a man is penetrated anally, pressure is put on the prostate gland (see illustration in chapter 3), which some men find highly pleasurable. Some women too describe intense feelings and even experience orgasm from being penetrated anally. While there is no scientific proof of this, some sex educators believe that when a woman is penetrated anally, pressure from the dildo or penis is put on her G-spot and this pressure is what is pleasuring her. It is also possible that the internal clitoral body is being stimulated.

> When I am tired and in pain but still feel like having sex, I like to lie on my stomach with pillows under my hips. This way I can still reach my clit with my good hand while my lover stimulates my anus. I make sure rubber gloves are used, with lots of lubricant. I love to feel the pressure of my body against the pillow with my hand between my legs. I like to take my time working on my fantasy while my lover whispers in my ear…it makes the fantasy even more real. When I'm really hot and wet my lover will slowly rub my asshole. He listens to my breathing…when it gets faster, he rubs a little harder and faster. Sometimes I try not to focus on one sensation but let it all run together until I come. Some of my orgasms have been total body releases, which often relieves the pain for a while.

Start slow, and take the time to explore. Pay attention to what feels good and what doesn't. If you start to experience negative feelings or if anything is painful or uncomfortable, stop what you are doing for a while. Just breathe and relax and then start again if you feel like it. Pain is a signal that helps protect you from injury. You should avoid experimenting with anal play if you are drunk or taking recreational drugs that may dull your senses. Anal sex does not have to hurt, and if it hurts you're doing it wrong. If you don't have anal sensation, then you will need to be particularly careful. In that case, in addition to using lots of extra lubricant, you may want to keep to smaller things for anal penetration.

Be creative and open your mind to all the possibilities of anal play. Some of them might involve playing with fingers or other body parts or objects, pulling open the buttocks (thereby stretching the anal opening), and penetration with fingers, toys, or penis. You can also take advantage of the fact that this is a taboo area for many of us. Anal play can inspire all sorts of rebellious or over-the-edge mental fantasies as well as verbal or nonverbal communication during the play itself.

Anal penetration can stimulate a bowel movement, especially for someone with little bowel control. So timing a bowel movement a few hours (or less) before this activity is a good idea.

The lining of the anus is very sensitive to damage so special precautions should be taken. Anything near or in the anus should be smooth and free of jagged edges. Using gloves is the easiest way to keep safe and clean. Otherwise be sure to cut your fingernails short, and round the edges with an emery board. If you are using dildos be sure to only use ones with a flared base. The rectum can create a vacuum effect and anything that slips out of your grasp may not be easily retrievable. Lubricant is essential for anal penetration as the anus does not produce its own lubrication.

Finally, keep clean. Do not put anything in the vagina that has been in the anus—bacteria that live quite happily in the anus can create serious problems in the vagina. If you are moving from the anus to the vagina, use a new condom on penis or toys and a new glove on hands, or wash very thoroughly. Use a dental dam or slice open a condom to use as a barrier for oral–anal contact to prevent the transmission of hepatitis and intestinal parasites.

Positions

A "good" position for sex is one that will let you do what you want to do, let you touch the parts of your partner or yourself that you want to touch, and let you be comfortable. So start thinking outside of the traditional positions you come across in movies, books, and television (all two of them!).

My favorite position is on my back with women. Of course it depends on what is going on: using a toy (I have used a toy with a man too, so it isn't limited as to what and where it can be used), caressing or rubbing her in various areas of her body, or her sitting on my face. It honestly depends on what she is into.

I definitely have favorite sexual positions. Because I have pain in my joints if they are used too much, stressed too much, or are in the wrong position too long, I find it easiest to be on my back with a long, cylindrical pillow under my knees and my partner over me. She and I like a lot of different things. We both like to kiss. I crave long, sexy kisses fully clothed in the kitchen (while burning the popcorn) as much as cunnilingus, vibrator play, petting, fisting, breast sucking, or strap-on fucking. But we find we can have almost all of those things in my best position. So we definitely have found ourselves in the same three positions (the others being one partner on hands and knees for fisting or fucking; and lesbian missionary—one of us on our back with the other lying between the first's legs instead of on top of her). In my most comfortable position, sometimes her toes are at the same end of the bed as mine, but sometimes we are facing in opposite directions. Does that make it two different positions? Possibly.

At first I am embarrassed to undress. Don't want a man to see my body. At my age, the body is not great anyway but added to my disability, it is not beautiful. I am tentative at first. So much depends on one's partner. I like any position I can manage!!!!

When I was with a mixed couple, it was on my back, legs pulled back, and her sitting on my face while he was doing my rear. But there were other positions that we got into, like lying on my stomach, side, and so on.

I rarely do the intercourse thing. I guess the positions that feel good are the ones where I'm being comfortably stimulated or am comfortably stimulating someone else. I love lying on my side kissing and hugging my lover—my left side is best to lie on so I can use my long right arm to touch them. I like sitting up and touching someone, but find it virtually impossible to sit on someone's face or torso without crushing them to death because of my short right leg. Some positions are definitely more comfortable than others. I rarely lie or climb on top of someone because I really can't support my own weight because of my disabilities.

I am very fortunate in that it is easy for me to achieve and sustain multiple orgasms within a relatively short period of time. If I chose to sleep with a man, my sex life would be made more difficult both because of my inability to spread my legs for prolonged periods of time and my increased spasticity upon sexual excitement. This generally interferes with the rhythm of heterosexual intercourse. During my one foray into heterosexual experience, I compensated for this difficulty by throwing my legs up over my head. My disability enables me to maintain this position comfortably and allows others to gain access to appropriate areas. Penetration is important but not essential.

Often we will try to adjust our needs to a particular position, when it would work better the other way around. So, for example, someone who is hemiplegic can lie on their affected side so that the unaffected arm is free to move. Frequently the solutions are simple, once you stop thinking that the missionary and doggie positions are the only way to have sex. Positioning is something you might be able to do on your own, or you may need to get your partner or an attendant to help (see chapter 4 for ideas on this kind of negotiation). Well-placed mirrors can help with positioning and also let you see yourself and your partner, which can be quite a turn-on. If you know you're likely to feel pain during sex, try to choose a position that allows you to move away easily if you're starting to experience pain.

Here are some tips that we have picked up over the years. You'll find more in chapter 7, on oral sex.

One Partner on Top

If you have a bad back, try lying on your back with pillows under your knees to keep your legs slightly bent. Some people also use a rolled-up towel under their lower back. This position can be used for almost any sexual activity. A variation on this is to lie on your front with a pillow under your hips or belly.

If one partner has more physical strength and control than the other, they may want to take a position on top with their partner lying on their back or side. While these positions are traditionally seen as top = superior, we want to suggest that the person on the bottom can have control of the action by saying exactly what they want and when.

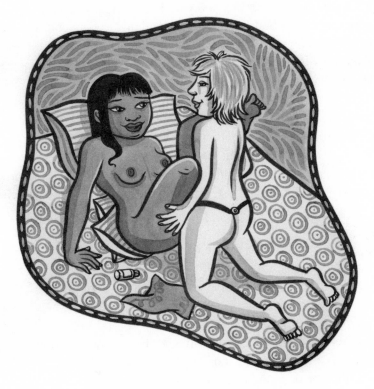

Illustration 7. Position: Partner on Top

Because of my disability I am unable to spread my legs without feeling a lot of pressure and pain in my hips. Being on top or on the bottom and lying on a flat surface like a bed isn't possible for me. What I have figured out is that if I lie on my back and hang my hips over the side of the bed or a couch, I can still have vaginal penetration. My partner kneels and then pulls me forward so my legs are straddling his hips and my bum is right on the edge of the bed. This way I can reach my clit and get fucked without feeling too much pressure or pain.

One partner can lie on their back with pillows for support. Their partner sits on top of them with legs on either side. If you have a good deal of upper body strength, you can do a lot being on top over your partner. If you spread your legs and your knees apart you can give room for the person on the bottom to move around underneath you. The partner on top can also work even if they can't move much below the waist. They can use their upper body to press against either the bed or their partner to create pelvic movement.

Or one partner can try lying on their back with their knees against their chest, or knees on their partner's shoulders. The other partner kneels facing the first partner. This position gives the person who is on their knees easy access for penetration, but the person on their back gets less movement. The person on their back can use their hands and arms for thrusting. If you can, you might also try squeezing your buttocks together.

Using Your Wheelchair

Sex in your wheelchair has the benefit of speed (if you don't have time for more than a quickie). You don't even need to get fully undressed!

A wheelchair with removable armrests can offer quite a few possibilities. Your partner can sit on your lap facing you with their legs on either side of you. In this position not only do you both have access to the whole top halves of your bodies to touch and feel and use for support, you can also touch and feel each other's bellies and upper thighs. If the person in the chair wants to penetrate their partner (with a penis or dildo), the partner can sit on the lap of the person in the chair, facing away for a rear entry position. They can use their arms to support themselves, leaning on your knees. They can also sit facing you with legs hanging down or wrapped around you, although this isn't comfortable for as long a period of time.

If your wheelchair doesn't have removable arms the position with your partner sitting on your lap facing away from you will likely be more comfortable. They then have the opportunity to use the armrests for support.

If the person in the wheelchair wants to be penetrated, they can use the same positions, with a partner sitting on top. For penetration or cunnilingus, they can scoot their butt (with or without help) forward in the chair and have the partner kneel or sit in front of the chair.

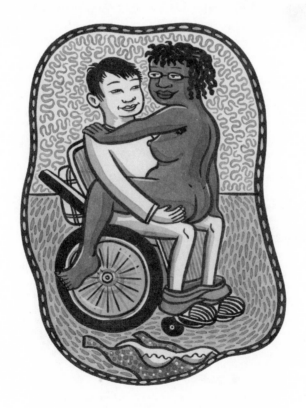

Illustration 8. Position: Using Wheelchair

Lying on Your Side

Lying side-to-side is an effective position for a person wearing a catheter attached to a leg bag. This gives you both room to move around and touch each other with many parts of your bodies.

People with hip problems who want to be penetrated can lie on their side with a pillow between their knees. In this position, they are penetrated from behind.

Side positions can also be used with partners facing each other. This position allows for either partner to provide the thusting movement (as opposed to one person on top of another, where the person on top needs to provide most of the movement).

With tight leg or hip tendons or muscles, one partner lies on their side. The other lies perpendicular to their partner with their knees bent

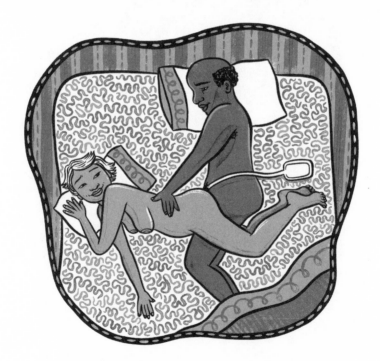

Illustration 9. Position: Side-by-Side

over their partner's waist. This position is very comfortable and can allow for longer, slower penetration sessions.

Using Furniture

Most people use furniture when having sex—most often, a bed. But here are other possibilities. One partner can kneel, with their upper body being supported by something (a bed, a comfy chair, plus some pillows). Their knees are on the ground (again with a pillow underneath them). The other partner can kneel behind them. This gives the partner from behind access to their partner's whole back, head, neck, and butt. But the partner being supported by the furniture has less access to their partner's body.

Or, one can partner sit on a couch or comfy chair. The other partner can sit between their legs, facing away from them.

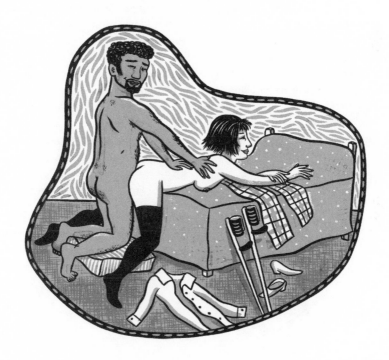

Illustration 10. Position: Using Furniture

PRODUCTS THAT HELP WITH POSITIONING

Some very old products, and one very new, have been designed to make sex positioning easier. They aren't designed specifically for penetration, and can be used for oral sex, masturbation, anal/vaginal penetration, or anything else.

The classic toy that is a boon for folks with all sorts of mobility and fatigue issues is the sling. There are about a dozen variations on the sling (some are made from leather, some from nylon; one of the newer ones is made of bungee cord material) but they all work on the same premise. They come with hardware and instructions to affix the sling to a ceiling, and they offer support that allows someone to sit or lie in the sling. This takes all the weight off the joints and limbs and allows for much more movement with a partner. A sling can be installed over a bed, so that even if neither partner is able to stand for long periods of time, one of them can be in the sling and the other can kneel or lie with pillows on the bed.

Over the years people have also manufactured pillows to assist in positioning. Regular pillows will do fine. But a new company has created a series of pillows in geometric shapes that are both versatile and firm, and ideal for sexual positioning. The only drawback to these products is that they are expensive and therefore out of reach for many of us. Some sex toy manufacturers make inflatable pillows that vibrate and are supposed to aid easier positioning. In our experience these plastic pillows are poor quality and are usually very uncomfortable to use (also they are not designed for larger folks and can break if too much weight is put on them). If you are thinking about buying one of these we recommend seeing it in person before putting your money down.

For information on where to find these products see Sexuality: Products (Toys, Books, Videos/DVDs) in chapter 14.

Sex Toys, Books, and Videos

I have found that sex isn't just getting an erection and wham, bang, thank you, ma'am. It is being able to share in good conversation, helping others cope with their own and overcoming my own inhibitions. I have also learned that getting an erection isn't that important, especially if you have a toy or two.

In this chapter we will answer some basic questions about sex toys and then discuss all the major kinds of toys, what they do and how to choose one toy over another. At the end of the chapter we'll discuss general adaptations to toys, safer sex with toys, and, if you've decided to buy a sex toy, how to access the best toys with the best service.

Who Uses Sex Toys?

Toys and tools are important, but they have their place with differ-
ent people and it is important to never force your partner into
something that they are not ready for. But if they are, take your
time and enjoy the feeling, using care and adaptive devices needed
to enable both to enjoy.

No one specific type of person uses sex toys. Bankers, cops, mothers,
grandfathers, religious people, and atheists all use them. Anyone you can
imagine may be the sort of person who uses sex toys. It's not that everyone is interested in sex toys, but that anyone might be. There just isn't a
sex-toy sort of person.

At the same time, sex toys are not for everyone. If you're not interested
in sex toys it doesn't mean there's something wrong with you, that you aren't
cool, or open enough, or that you're missing out on the best sex of your life.
Far from it: Sex toys are only good when their use is something that feels right
for you. All we want to suggest is that everyone has the right to experimentation and choice in their sex lives. And this includes the right to play with
sex toys, as much as it includes the right to have no interest at all in them.

Why Use Sex Toys?

People use sex toys for a huge variety of reasons. Sex toys can be fun.
They provide pleasure. Some people need strong and consistent stimulation to get off, and some sex toys will provide this. Sex toys can change
the nature or content of fantasy during solo sex as well as with other people. They can be tools of self-assertion. Sex toys can do things humans
can't. Sex toys are goofy and can make you laugh.

Sex Toys as Tools of Empowerment

Sexual independence is an extremely powerful form of empowerment
that permeates all aspects of our lives. One of us has been selling sex toys

for the past fifteen years. It feels political and slightly revolutionary, and it's unbelievably gratifying to be playing a small part in individual revolutions that are taking place all over the world.

How is all this possible from a small vibrating object (to give just one example of a sex toy)? The most revolutionary aspect of sex toys is that they let us do things for ourselves. When we please ourselves, controlling what happens on our own terms, we are engaging in truly radical sex. Consider the fact that we have often been told that giving someone pleasure is more important than giving it to ourselves. A great lover, the myth has it, is always defined by the heights of passion they can take someone else to, never by the ingenious ways they can pleasure themselves. The flip side of this is that we are only supposed to feel pleasure when it's given to us as a gift from someone else (one of the reasons why masturbation is seen as second-class sex). At the risk of sounding selfish, we think this is nonsense. A great lover, in our view, is someone who knows how to please himself or herself, someone who is comfortable with himself or herself, and is willing to take the risk of sharing that experience with someone else.

Sex toys are also tools of self-assertion, in that they will never ask you to do something you don't want to do. No dildo or vibrator is ever going to coerce you into a sexual encounter. This is one of the reasons so many therapists recommend sex toys to people who have experienced sexual abuse and are trying to come back to trusting sex with other people.

Sex toys allow us to empower ourselves through three processes that often occur before we have a toy we can play with:

- Asserting one's right to feel pleasure
- Facilitating improved communication
- Furthering our self-understanding.

First, we have to acknowledge a desire. If you buy yourself a sex toy, you do so to please yourself. You are making a statement that you are interested in feeling pleasure, and you are worthy of that pleasure. This is no small achievement, and it's one of the reasons so many of us feel unsure about talking about sex toys. It can be hard to say (with our actions), "I am worthy of pleasure. This does not make me needy or selfish."

The next step involves getting information about sex toys. Where do you turn if you want to know something about vibrators, for example? Finding out can be quite a bit of work for people who don't have private access to the Internet. Often people start by asking a friend, partner, doctor, coworker. This first question is another bold move. Most of us want the opportunity to talk about sex: to ask our questions, to share our fears, to laugh about how silly it is sometimes. By taking that risk and starting the conversation, we are opening ourselves up to new possibilities for communication. In our experience most people want the chance to talk about sex and are thankful when someone else makes the first move.

BECOMING ADDICTED TO SEX TOYS

A common question about sex toys is whether you can become addicted to them. The short answer is no. Wanting to do something often does not mean that you are addicted. We don't talk about people being addicted to breathing or sleeping. There is nothing harmful about safely using sex toys, even if you use them often. You can get very different things from a sex toy and a person. You can't have a conversation with a sex toy. On the other hand, it will never say, "I have a headache." Discovering vibrators and the sensations they produce can be somewhat intoxicating. At first, we may use the vibrator a lot, perhaps masturbating much more than before. If this makes you worried or anxious, you could set a time limit to just go nuts with it (a couple of weeks or a month perhaps) and then reexamine your use, see if it is interfering with other things you would like to or should be doing, and if so, just back down a bit. It is true that you can become used to the feel of sex toys and find that other things don't turn you on as they used to. People can get into a "sexual rut" where we do the same thing over and over again and stop trying new things. This doesn't happen just with sex toys. If you are worried about relying on sex toys, go back to a kind of sex you were having before, or try something brand new. With a little bit of time and patience you'll rediscover a love for other ways of turning yourself on. No negative effects have been documented of playing safely with sex toys.

Finally, you have to get the courage to actually buy a sex toy (you can take books from a library, and rent videos, but no one rents sex toys). In a big city you will probably be able to find a store where the workers are positive about sex and the customers they serve. If you pick a store at random, or if you live in a smaller town, you may end up with staff who are bored and not very knowledgeable. As always, access is likely to be an issue. Luckily many excellent companies offer paper catalogs through the mail, and online catalogs are readily available on the Internet (for names and addresses see chapter 14).

Once you have the toy, you can use it. Most people will try out their sex toy by themselves, without a partner. The freedom from having to focus on a partner gives you the opportunity to concentrate on yourself. Focusing on yourself and, with luck, having a little more time to explore gives you the opportunity to discover the more subtle aspects of your sexual response, such as the small areas that drive you wild and little movements that get you over the top. You may also discover what you aren't comfortable with. This too furthers self-understanding.

Sex toys are also reminders of the diversity of sexual expression and are also potential levelers, as they offer the same services to anyone who uses them.

Other Reasons to Try Sex Toys

Trying something new is another reason to consider a sex toy. We may already be completely satisfied with our sexual activities alone and with partners. Trying new things is often thought to be kinky, or dangerous. But if you really like a particular kind of food, say cheese, you will want to try different kinds of cheeses, to broaden your tastes and horizons. When it comes to sex, if you are happy with what you've got, is it considered wrong to check out other options? Wanting to experiment with sex toys may be just for the interest of experimenting.

For many people a vibrator is the first (and the easiest) way to experience an orgasm. Nothing moves like a vibrator—no hand, no penis, no elbow, nothing. Many women can have an orgasm from other kinds of stimulation once they have learned to have an orgasm from a vibrator.

Each man will respond to different intensities of stimulation. A vibrator can broaden the experience of being stimulated erotically. For some men a vibrator will be strong enough stimulation to have an orgasm.

We know that the more times a woman experiences a sexual response the more reliable her response becomes. Climaxes bring more climaxes. For men a similar situation exists in terms of understanding and control of response. The more a man can play with himself sexually, be playful and mindful of what gives him pleasure, the greater understanding and sensitivity he can have in terms of his actual response (that is, excitement leading to climax) as well as the limitless ways he can feel pleasure. In all of this we're not just talking about orgasms. It may be that a climax for you is something other than an orgasm you experienced before, or the orgasms you think you should be having. Sex toys can open you up to your potential and help you find your own sexual climax.

What Are Sex Toys?

I have this feather duster that I bought in Chinatown. I brush it lightly over my breasts and belly. Most of the time it drives me wild, but sometimes it just tickles, I don't know why.

I keep looking for the perfect dildo, not too long or too short, not too fat or too skinny, firm but not hard, attractive to look at. I haven't found this all in one sex toy yet, but I'm still looking. I think I'll start taking measurements with me when I go shopping. At the store I get turned on looking at dildos that are bigger that what I actually want. I think they look perfect but then when I go home and try it it just isn't right.

My best thing for sex is a hose that attaches to my bathtub faucet. It came with a shower head kind of thing but I threw that out. I love feeling the pressure of the water on my clit.

Two old terms for sex toys that we emphatically *don't* use are *sexual aids* and *marital aids*. You don't need to be married to want to use sex toys (to which the three of us say, thank goodness!). The term *aid* implies that the toy is a replacement or an assistive device, which it isn't. Assistive devices are created by people who know what they're doing, and often a lot of thought is put into them. Unfortunately, sex toys are usually made by people who haven't thought very much about how they will be used. The majority of them are mass manufactured and have never been tested at all. Sex toys may function as assistive devices, but they haven't been thoughtfully designed as such. For this reason we don't like the term *sexual aid*. It's important to be realistic about the limitations of the products.

The best parallel we've come up with is that a sex toy is like a child's teddy bear. A teddy can provide great comfort, a sense of security, warmth, and can even be sort of sexy to sleep with. But it isn't a replacement for being tucked in by parents, or being hugged or kissed goodnight, or playing with friends. It provides something entirely different. Sex toys aren't meant to be replacements for interpersonal relationships, nor do they make you never want to have sex with other people. They provide something completely different; they are just toys for adults.

A towel can be a sex toy. A paintbrush might be a sex toy. Or a store-bought vibrator, erotic movie, or smutty book can be a sex toy.

Imagination and our ability to fantasize is the most diverse, multipurpose sex toy there is—and it's free. You'll never find a premade sex toy that will be as interesting as what you can create in your mind. Sex toys are animated not by incredible design, but really by our imaginations (plus sometimes a couple of AA batteries!).

Beyond the gift of fantasy, though, you have at your command a number of basic kinds of sex toys. The rest of this chapter is divided into a discussion of each of these kinds of toys, ways to use them and adapt them to your needs. Following the description of each sex toy we have included a very rough estimate of its cost (in U.S. dollars).

Vibrators

> *Masturbation is very important to me. It used to be a lot easier.*
> *I could cum by fucking my urinal. As I've gotten a lot older it is much*
> *more difficult to masturbate. About a year and a half ago I found a*
> *vibrator I can use. It is very strong; I'm not very gentle on things and I*
> *tend to break everything. It is electric so there are no batteries to worry*
> *about. It has an on/off switch that is strong enough for me to use. The*
> *switch is fairly large and not stiff. The vibrating head is very big, there-*
> *fore, if I can get it close to the right spot, that's close enough. Setting*
> *up is a nonissue for me as I employ my own attendants. I know that it*
> *wouldn't be possible in all the other services I've had in the past.*

Vibrators are probably the best known of all sex toys. They can be separated into two main categories: electric (or plug-in) models, and battery-powered models.

Electric Vibrators

You can find electric vibrators in big department stores near the hair dryers. They are packaged as "massagers" and the boxes feature pictures of people using the massager almost everywhere above the waist. There is never an indication that the "massager" can be used below the waist or for anything other than muscle relaxation. These are the same massagers often used in rehab clinics for all kinds of physical therapy work. The secret that the manufacturers and rehab professionals don't mention is that they can feel great and are perfectly safe on all parts of our bodies.

Electric vibrators are the best quality vibrators available. They usually come with warranties and are made by large, relatively reputable companies. They also provide much stronger vibrations than most battery-operated models. The drawbacks to electric vibrators are that they are larger, heavier, and more unwieldy than other toys. They tend to be more expensive and often are only for external stimulation and cannot be used for penetration (though now a few companies are making attachments for electric vibrators that you can use for penetration).

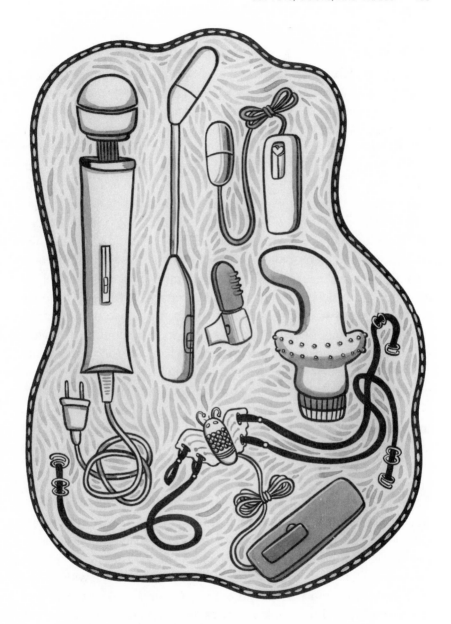

Illustration 11. Vibrators

Electric vibrators come in two kinds: coil vibrators and wand vibrators. The coil electric vibrator is almost silent when it is on because it doesn't have a motor that whirrs. Instead the vibration is created by an electro-magnetic coil inside the case of the vibrator. These vibrators usually come with a variety of attachments. Coil vibrators have a more pointed vibration, and though they are not as strong as the vibrations that come from wand type vibrators they may feel more intense. Because of their smaller size and shape, coil vibrators are most effective when they can be held with one (or two) hands. Another limitation with this design is that the attachments tend to be small, offering a smaller vibrating surface, which may make it difficult to get it exactly where you want it and keep it there.

The more popular and common model of electric vibrator is the wand massager. These vibrators are usually ten to twelve inches in length with a large head that vibrates. They make more noise but are stronger and have the benefit of a larger vibrating surface. Because of this they are usually more adaptable, as they can fit between two people or rest beside one person, and still "hit" the right spot. Some wand vibrators have a curved handle, which makes them easier to reach with. Wand style vibrators usually have two speeds. Some need to be plugged in each time, while others are rechargeable and come with an adapter to do this. The benefit of the rechargeable vibrators is that you don't need to be near a plug to use it. The drawback is that the charge may run out at the worst possible time! Electric vibrators range in price anywhere from $40 to $200.

Battery-Powered Vibrators

The more common type of vibrator for use as a sex toy is the battery-powered model. They provide a gentler vibration than electric vibrators. The benefits of battery-powered vibrators are that they are quieter, lighter weight, and less expensive, plus they come in a much wider range of shapes, sizes, and colors. The drawback is that they are usually of poorer quality and don't last nearly as long as electric models. A few differences exist among battery-powered vibrators: material, quality of motor, and shape/size/color.

Hard plastic vibrators usually provide stronger stimulation than the soft ones and are easier to clean. But they tend to be louder, and can crack if dropped. Hard plastic toys sometimes have seams that must be filed down before use. A lot of people prefer hard plastic toys just for external stimulation and use soft rubber vibrators for penetration.

Soft rubber toys are quieter than the hard ones and usually have milder vibration. Most people find them more comfortable for penetration play. They are also more durable as they are unlikely to crack if dropped. A major drawback with soft rubber toys is that they are more difficult to get clean and keep clean because the material is usually porous. Sometimes the material will break down before the motor does. One kind of soft rubber we'll talk more about later is called silicone rubber. Silicone is a much cleaner,

> **THINGS TO THINK ABOUT WHEN CHOOSING A VIBRATOR**
>
> 1. Do you want something for just external stimulation, something for penetration, or both?
> 2. If you're looking for something for penetration, do you want something you can use vaginally or anally, or both?
> 3. What about shape, size, color? Do you want something that looks and feels like a cock, or something completely nonrepresentational?
> 4. Some vibrators you hold on to, and others you can strap to your body. Which would you prefer?
> 5. What material do you want?
> 6. How much do you want to spend? We suggest starting with less expensive vibrators if it's your first time, but less expensive usually means it won't last as long.

durable form of rubber that will last longer. Silicone also has the benefit of transmitting vibrations very well, thus toys made from silicone tend to feel stronger.

Another practical difference among battery-powered vibrators is the quality of the motor. Most vibrators are made with very cheap Chinese motors that burn out easily. Some toys are made with higher quality Japanese motors. These are more expensive, but last longer and feel better. Often the only way to know what kind of motor is in a toy is to ask. Sometimes staff won't know the answer. We recommend only buying toys from companies that can provide you with answers to questions like these. If you are in a store, you can ask to see the package and check where the toy is made.

Battery-powered toys vary widely in price. An inexpensive battery-powered vibrator can be $9 and a silicone toy with a Japanese motor can be as much as $150.

Dildos

A dildo is a toy that doesn't vibrate and is designed mainly for penetration. Depending on the shape, a dildo may be safe for vaginal penetration, anal

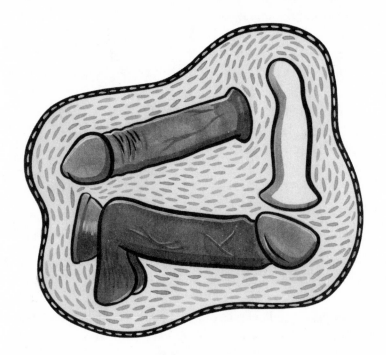

Illustration 12. Dildos

penetration, or both. Some people also get pleasure from how a dildo looks, whether on its own, inserted in you, or being worn by yourself or someone else with a harness. Dildos are made from a variety of materials, including rubber, glass, wood, plastic, and leather. Every material has its benefits and drawbacks. Your choice should be based on what you want to do with it, what will work best for you, and personal taste. In general, a firmer dildo, or one with a good curve, will be better for G-spot stimulation for women and prostate stimulation for men. Firmer dildos are also easier to use in harnesses. The look and shape of the dildo is quite important for some people. Some dildos are surprisingly realistic-looking and - feeling, modeled from real penises and complete with veins and balls that move. For people who are turned off by realistic-looking penises there are dildos that look like dolphins, goddesses, cats, or nothing in particular.

THE PLAIN RUBBER VS. SILICONE RUBBER CONTROVERSY

Many of the higher-end sex toy stores have ongoing debates about whether it is safe to recommend and use plain rubber dildos. Some people say that the cheaper rubber is of unknown origin and has many chemicals and dyes that eventually leach out and into our bodies. These people often say that silicone is the only material to put in your body. We can think of two problems with this argument. First, no scientific studies have been conducted on this. We simply don't know if the claims of harm are true. We do know that people have been using cheap rubber toys for years and there has yet to be any major health crisis related to it. Second, many of us will never be able to afford $80 for a sex toy. That said, the most balanced of sex stores seem to go with the following advice: Silicone is a very safe material to use, but if you are using less expensive rubber dildos, and you have concerns about their safety, always use a condom on the toy. Using condoms won't change the way most toys feel, and they are also a great way to keep the toy clean and extend its life span. Maybe one day "60 Minutes" will investigate, but until then we all have to assess the risk for ourselves and choose what to do. We only caution you against being talked into a more expensive toy than you want. You can always find ways to play safe and cheap!

The best-quality soft rubber dildos available are made with silicone rubber. Silicone is ideal for sex toys. It retains temperature much better than plain rubber, so it will heat up to your body temperature as you use it. It is a much cleaner form of rubber, it tends to be hypoallergenic, and because silicone can withstand high temperatures, you can clean your silicone toys by boiling them in water for three to five minutes. Silicone also comes in a much wider range of color choices. Because silicone toys are handmade by small manufacturers, it is easier to find out information about the material if you have specific allergies or sensitivities. The main drawback to silicone is that it is usually twice the price of plain rubber. Plain rubber dildos range from $12 to $40, while silicone toys range from $50 to $150.

Anal Toys

Anything used for anal penetration should have a flared base, large enough so that the toy can't slip into the rectum. The rectum can create a vacuum effect, and objects that don't have a big base can quickly be drawn up into your body. While it is true that what goes up will come down eventually, we don't recommend you take that chance. To play safe, only use a toy with a flared base, one with a large handle, or one with some sort of ring on the end that will prevent the toy from slipping all the way in.

People use three kinds of toys for anal play. The first are dildos with flared bases. People usually use these toys for penetration with some variation on an in/out motion. If you use a curved dildo it is easier to stimulate the prostate for men.

The second most common anal toy is called a butt plug. Butt plugs are small at the tip, gradually get wider, and then get small again just before the flared base. The benefit of these toys is that once inserted, they will stay in much better than a regular dildo. People will insert a butt plug (or have someone else do it) as part of sex play and then do other things while the plug is in. It is perfectly safe to leave a butt plug in for a while as long as you're able to monitor your own sensations around the anus (see safer sex tips later in this chapter for more ideas on this). Both dildos and butt plugs can come in vibrating and nonvibrating styles. Many vibrating anal toys come with Chinese motors, and some are made with the better quality Japanese motors.

The third kind of anal toy is anal beads. Sometimes called Thai beads, these are a series of five or six round hard plastic or soft rubber beads attached by a stout string or cord. The idea is that the beads are inserted slowly, with lots of lubricant, and then slowly pulled out. Unlike dildos and plugs, the pleasure from the toy doesn't come from having it inside, but instead from the sensation as they pass along the two ringed sphincter muscles. If you are using hard plastic anal beads it is very important to check for seams before you use them the first time. If there are seams they should be filed down with an emery board before first

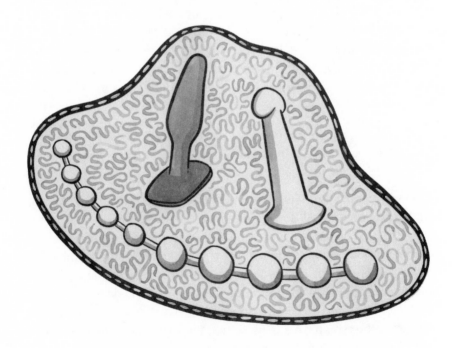

Illustration 13. Anal Toys

use. Another problem with beads is keeping the string or cord clean. Most of these beads cannot be boiled in water, and the string is usually cotton or nylon. Nylon string is best. But better yet, several styles of anal beads are entirely made of jelly rubber with no string at all. They still can't be boiled, but rubber is much less absorbent than string and these kinds of beads will last longer. Toys are a way to start exploring the pleasure potential of this area with less stress than trying to negotiate anal play with a partner. The price of anal toys varies based on the kind of toy and the material. Plugs can be as low as $8, and beads are usually also inexpensive (even the best ones should be under $30).

Harnesses

A harness allows you to use a dildo with someone else without having to hold on to it. The most popular harnesses are waist harnesses, which go around the waist and have one or two straps designed to go between the legs. Other harnesses let you strap a dildo around your thigh, or around your arm (even around your chin), and a third category of harness is designed to let you strap a dildo onto something else (see sidebar).

> *Penetration is only important for those I am with, because I can't get an erection. But in my mind I do like to insert the dildo and see and feel my partner enjoy it.*

Many people use harnesses to penetrate a partner with a dildo without holding on to it. All sorts of people use harnesses in this way—men who can't always get an erection, but like to penetrate their partners; women who want to penetrate their (male or female) partners; men who can get erections but choose to try something different. Harnesses also facilitate fantasy play. When you strap on a harness and dildo you are not only strapping on a new body part, you can also strap on a different persona. Whether you have a penis or not, playing with the fantasy of having this new penis (which may be a very different shape and feel from your own, or may be entirely new if you've never had one) can be exhil-

AN ACCESSIBLE TOY STORY

A frustrating idea that nondisabled people often have is that to make something accessible is difficult, expensive, and just a general pain in the ass. While this usually isn't true (except in people's heads), there is no question that it is much easier to make something accessible from its creation than to go back and change it later. Most sex toys aren't very accessible. They have ridiculous designs; they are made for a small percentage of the population in terms of the array of people's needs and physical abilities. But with only a few small modifications in design it doesn't have to be that way. A perfect example is an ingenious toy made by a San Francisco–based company called Stormy Leather. The toy is called the Night Rider. The Night Rider is essentially like any other thigh harness. It is designed to let you strap a dildo on to something. The problem with most thigh harnesses is that the straps are made for people with only certain size thighs (which quickly excludes anyone without thighs also). The folks at Stormy Leather fixed this problem by making the Night Rider with just under five feet of strapping. Thus their toy can go around any size thigh, not to mention a wheelchair, a (small) tree, anything. The cost of adding this extra length is minimal and the toy's retail cost is about the same as most thigh harnesses. It's a perfect example of a toy that is adaptable and didn't require space age modifications. Most manufacturers don't think about accessibility. But some small manufacturers have expressed interest in making more accessible toys. If you're interested in offering suggestions, see the Sexuality: Products (Toys, Books, Videos/DVDs) section of chapter 14 on sex toy resources.

arating, freeing, and a fascinating way to explore gender. This is to say nothing of the fun your new penis can give you and your partner. Harnesses range in price depending on the material and durability. Inexpensive harnesses can start at $40, with most running from $60 to $100.

Toys for Men

Men can use almost any kind of sex toy. Dildos and vibrators are marketed for women but are just as much fun for men. Some toys are made specifically for penises. They can be divided into three groups: insertion toys, cock rings, and pumps.

Insertion toys are designed to have a penis inserted into them. The main difference in these toys is whether or not they vibrate.

A whole host of nonvibrating insertion toys are available for men. These are usually cylindrical toys that have a hole running through the shaft that is designed to be penetrated by a penis. Some are made to look like body parts (vagina, anus, mouth), and others aren't supposed to look like anything at all. You can consider all of them to provide an alternative to the feeling of a human hand, mouth, ass, vagina, or whatever. Most of these toys require that you or someone else hold on to them, and for most people the pleasure comes from moving them up and down the shaft of the penis. Some toys even have "ribs" inside that provide extra stimulation.

Vibrating toys offer a completely different sensation. Most toys of this type look the same as the nonvibrating toys but have a vibrator either on the outside of the cylinder or somewhere inside the rubber. Some of these toys provide strong stimulation and a nice feeling. If you are looking for a toy like this, be aware of where the vibrator is placed. The best place is at the opening, where the penis goes in. That way the vibrator can stimulate whatever part of your penis you prefer. If the vibrator is placed deep inside the toy it probably won't work as well. In terms of cleanup, a lot of these toys are not open ended, so if you ejaculate into the toy it's almost impossible to get it fully clean. The best designs are those that are hollow all the way through, allowing for easy cleanup. Some vibrating toys will stay on the penis, allowing you to have vibration without having to hold the toy, yet others are too floppy to stay on and require at least one hand, if not two hands, to use them. All these toys require you to use a lubricant with them, as the rubber is always dry and often sticky. Insertion toys for men vary in price from $30 to $100 depending on the quality of the material and whether there is vibration or not.

The second group of sex toys for men is *cock rings*. A cock ring is a piece of material (usually rubber or leather) that goes around the base of the penis and behind the scrotum. Men use cock rings for different reasons. For men with genital sensation they can be a pleasurable toy in themselves. They create a feeling of warmth and pressure and focus your attention on your genitals in a new and different way. Some men also wear rings because they like the way they make their genitals look. Some men, regardless of genital sensation, say that rings allow them to maintain an erection. A ring will not give you an erection, but if you have one, the ring works by holding blood in the penis, thus maintaining the erection. They don't work for everyone, and they don't always work each time. Rings differ in the way they go on and come off. The easiest rings to use have Velcro fasteners. These can be taken off with very little effort. The most difficult rings to use are ones that are solid rubber and not very stretchy. Note an important safety rule: Cock rings should not be used for more than thirty minutes at a time. Rings work by temporarily restricting the flow of blood out of the penis, and blood flow should not be restricted for more than thirty minutes. Setting a timer can help with this. If you think it may be difficult for you to get the ring off, allow for extra time or have someone around who can help you. Cock rings range in price from $10 to $30.

The third group of sex toys is *penis pumps*. The ads for pumps seem to promise a permanently enlarged penis, an erection whenever you want it, and a dream home in Barbados. All of these are far from the truth. The way a penis pump works is simple: The pump goes over the penis and has to be held tightly against the body. Pumping draws air out of the cylinder, creating a vacuum. This pulls blood into the penis, leading to an erection (barring circulatory problems). Once the pump is removed, if the man isn't aroused, or if he has problems maintaining erections, the erection will go away. Both men and women also use pumps as a sensation toy on other parts of the body (often the nipples and clitoris, but you can use them anywhere). By drawing blood to the surface of the skin covered by the pump you can create different sensations that some find pleasurable. Pumps range in price, anywhere from $30 to $300. We want to caution you that pumps are the most lied-about product (by manufacturers and many retailers) and, as a result, often the most disappointing toy people try. If you're interested in trying a pump out, be sure to start with an inexpensive one. They may not work as well as the higher-end pumps, but they should give you an idea of whether you like the feeling and the effect of the pump on your body. Several conditions may make pump use ill advised: any kind of peripheral vascular disease, blood clotting disorders, or diabetes. You should also not use a pump if you are taking blood thinning medication. If you have any concerns about using a pump we suggest you talk to a professional whom you trust and know won't be freaked out by sex questions.

Several medical devices are penis pumps with a series of cock rings. These devices have been clinically tested and are of better quality than the pumps and rings available in sex stores. The combination creates and then maintains an erection. They tend to cost several hundred dollars and in many countries require a prescription from a doctor.

Lubricants

Lube is the great unsung sex toy. Lubricants make everything feel nicer. Whether you're playing with yourself or with a partner, using toys or using body parts, lube makes everything more slippery. Lack of lubrication can make penetration or even genital touching painful. Natural lubrication can be reduced because of medications, hormonal changes, or decreased interest in sex. The first distinction in lubricants is whether they are water-based, oil-based, or silicone-based. Most lubricants that you can buy in sex stores or drugstores are water-based. These lubricants contain no oils that will harm latex, and are also easily flushed out of the body. Oil-based lubricants (which are rarer these days) will damage condoms and will also damage your rubber toys over time. Also, some people suggest that oil-based products are less likely to fully flush out of your body and can increase your chances of getting a bacterial infection. Silicone-based lubricants feel a lot like oil (they don't dry up) but are safe for use with condoms. However, the people who worry about oil-based lubes say the same concern goes for silicone-based lubes. To get oil or silicone lubes completely off your body, you need to use soap and water.

One other caution with silicone-based lubricants is to never use them with silicone toys as they will destroy them even with only a little bit of contact. You may see the term *water-soluble* used to describe a lube. This just means it will break down in water, and won't stain your sheets. It doesn't mean it contains no oils, and so there is a chance it will damage condoms and rubber toys.

The Feel of Lubricant

The consistency of lubricant varies from almost like water to thick as Jell-O. One is not necessarily better than the other, they are just different. You may want to consider what kind of lube would be easiest for you to use. If it takes you some time to get your hand from the bottle of lube to where you want the lube to be, a really slippery lube that slides right off your hand will be no good; a thicker lube might be easier. By contrast, thin lube will slide down your body quite well. If you are in an upright position you can pour the lube down your body (having it end up where you want it). Most people find thicker lube easier for anal play.

How Long the Lubricant Lasts

The water in water-based lubricants evaporates as they are applied and used, leaving a slightly tacky feeling and no lubrication. When this happens you don't need to apply more lube, you can just add some water (or saliva) to reinvigorate the lubricant. One exception to this is Liquid Silk, a British product that boasts a "nontacky" formulation. When Liquid Silk dries up it feels more like a moisturizer. One drawback to this lube is that it has a distinctly bitter taste.

There hasn't been much in the way of proper testing to see which lubricant lasts longer. Every company says theirs lasts the longest and you can read two magazines that did tests and find two different answers. Currently the longest-lasting lubricants that are safe for use with condoms seem to be the silicone-based products. Because they contain no water they don't dry up like water-based lubes. The best thing is to try out different kinds of lubricants to see which work best for you.

What Is in the Lubricants?

One final distinction between lubricants is their ingredients. It's very important to know what is in anything you use on or in your body. While most of us know this for food, clothing, and medication, we tend to forget it when it comes to sex toys.

Finding accurate information about the possible side effects of ingredients in lubricants is difficult. While there is little research, the three main concerns in terms of ingredients seem to be glycerin, methyl or propyl paraben, and nonoxynol-9.

Glycerin is a sweet-tasting fat byproduct that makes lube slippery. Many sex educators have suggested that people prone to yeast infections should avoid lubricants with glycerin. Slippery Stuff and Liquid Silk are two lubricants that contain no glycerin.

Almost all lubricants use methyl or propyl paraben as a preservative. Some people have allergic reactions to this ingredient. If you do, or suspect you might, it would be best to avoid lubricants that use it.

Thankfully fewer and fewer companies are putting the spermicide nonoxynol-9 in lubicants and lubricated condoms. This is a very harsh detergent and many people react to it. We strongly recommend avoiding lubricants with this ingredient.

Unfortunately, very few big manufacturers make lubricants with natural preservatives. The oldest and most popular one is called Probe, which uses grapefruit seed extract instead of methyl paraben. The manufacturer has an 800 number that you can call to find out where to purchase Probe near you. See the Sexuality: Products section of chapter 14.

For some people the taste of the lube is an issue. Some lubricants have a slightly sweet taste, some have a bitter taste, a few have no taste at all. Many companies also make flavored lubricants (cherry, strawberry, and others). Unfortunately, many of these seem to contain NutraSweet as a sugar substitute. Some people are concerned that NutraSweet may have negative health effects, and if you are one of them you may want to stay away from these. There is no solid scientific evidence that small amounts of this additive are harmful. Many lubricants are available in little trial-size packets for $1. Bottles of lubricant range in price depending on how much is in the bottle. Generally prices range from $8 to $30.

Sensation Toys

Toys designed to stimulate the five senses are called *sensation toys*. Many of these would be considered to be S/M toys but can be used in other ways (see chapter 11 for a more detailed discussion of this). The feather duster described earlier in the chapter would be a sensation toy. Ice cubes could also fit into this category.

> *I am heavily into S/M. I have been able to purchase ankle and arm restraints made out of leather. Steel handcuffs or other restraints could really hurt me due to my uncontrollable spasms.*

Sensation toys can be divided into toys for bondage, toys for flagellation or percussion, and clamps.

The most common toys for *bondage* are restraints. Restraints can be used to restrain a person (or some body part) during sex play. They come in a variety of materials, colors, and styles. The best kind is of a material that won't dig into the body (soft leather, fabric, soft rubber). It is also important to consider the way the restraint goes on and comes off, to make sure you can get out of them easily and quickly if necessary. Of course you can use all sorts of things to restrain someone (stockings, nightgown belt, silk tie). It is important to make sure that when you restrain someone the object you use isn't going to be cutting off their circulation or otherwise cutting into their skin.

People also use toys like collars and blindfolds as a form of bondage. By completely removing one sense (in this case sight) blindfolds impose a form of bondage on the individual. Many people find this sensory deprivation can heighten awareness of other senses. Collars can also be used to restrain someone or can simply symbolize in the moment that one person is being dominated, led around either literally or figuratively, by their partner. Collars should not be tight and should never be pulled from behind.

The other major category of toys are ones used for *flagellation and percussion* (defined as some kind of "hitting"). These include paddles, whips, floggers, canes, and feathers, each creating a unique sensation—from soft and enveloping, to harsh and stinging, to ticklish. Some people may scream with delight and squirm in ecstasy from the touch of a feather, while others wouldn't notice a tickle from a dozen feathers, and want stronger stimulation.

Another popular sensation toy is *nipple clamps*. These come in a variety of styles, each designed to stay on the nipple, creating an experience of pain and heightened awareness. Each kind has some sort of surface that goes on either side of the nipple and then a mechanism for adjusting the tension. Some styles are easier to manipulate than others, and some are more adjustable than others. With clamps there is an initial sensation when they are applied. This may be large or small depending on the tension of the clamp. Once the clamps have been on for a while the feeling usually subsides. It is when the clamps are removed that the most intense rush of sensation comes as blood rushes back to the nipple, and removing the clamps quickly or slowly will change the kind of sensation you feel. Don't fall asleep with nipple clamps on, as prolonged use can interfere with the blood supply to the nipples.

Massage Oils, Creams, Lotions

Oils, creams, and lotions can be used as part of sex play. Plain massage oils tend to be scented but not flavored and are made for full body massage and external use only. Brands that are made for professional masseurs tend to be of higher quality and are better for people with sensitive skin or environmental sensitivities. As a general rule, the cheesier the packaging the more crap will be in the product (look at the ingredient list, though, as this rule doesn't always work).

Warming oils contain glycerin and feel like they get hotter when massaged in or blown on. They create the sensation of heat without making your skin temperature go up. These products are usually edible and flavored and are not made for full body massage but rather for playing around on small parts of the body. Most edible products are like fast food: You should be sure to check the ingredient list before covering yourself or a loved one with these products!

Other products promise to "do" things: create arousal, make nipples tingle, tighten a vagina, or make a penis hard for hours. In general we recommend staying away from all these products. Most of them have never been approved for use as a cosmetic or for consumption as food. Arousal creams don't do what they say they will and may cause skin rashes or urinary tract infections.

The products that offer delayed ejaculation for men are similarly problematic. All these products (Sta-hard, Stud 100, Maintain, China Brush, and many more) merely use a local anesthetic to diminish sensation. By interfering with arousal, they delay ejaculation. The problems with this are obvious. Not only do they diminish pleasure, they also send the message that an erection is the only way for men to give and receive pleasure. We know and you know this isn't true. These creams remove men from their body responses. Good sex and feeling sexual have to come from within, from feeling pleasure. Desensitizing creams and sprays tell us, "Don't worry about your body, just perform."

Products that are called Spanish Fly or offer some sort of promise of arousal can be harmful. Most such products contain a natural or chemical bladder irritant. When someone takes the pill or liquid they may notice that they feel different "down there." What the manufacturer calls arousal is actually bladder irritation that may make the bladder more susceptible to infection. These products should be avoided completely.

Books

We've already said that the brain is the most important sexual organ, so it makes sense that we think books can serve as sex toys.

TIPS ON CHOOSING AN EROTIC BOOK

- Do you think you'd prefer short stories, or a novel? The benefit of an anthology of short stories is that if you hate one story you usually have another twenty to go.
- Think about the kind of sex you want to read about. Many anthologies are based on a theme (lesbian, gay, S/M, African American, and so on).
- How raunchy do you want to get? Do you want soft romance books that only hint at the action, or books that are wall-to-wall, head-board-pounding sex?
- Since most libraries don't carry good erotica, consider getting a few people together who can each buy a book and then you can swap.
- If you've never read any sex books, we suggest you start with an anthology that covers a lot of ground (different people, multiple kinds of sex, various settings). That way you can get an idea of what you might like and you aren't limiting your options.

Sexually explicit material (called *erotica* or *pornography*) has a number of uses. It can be entertaining and arousing. It can help us expand our fantasy abilities. Many people have not developed their fantasy lives, particularly those who lacked good access to sexual health education and sex material while growing up. Reading erotica can be an excellent way to expand your sexual fantasy repertoire and make up for some of those early losses. It provides us with scenarios, language, and imagery that we can take and make our own.

Erotic material has never been easier to access. Whether online, in mainstream bookstores, or in magazines, erotica has become a huge industry and is far more accepted and acceptable than in the past. However, it is hard to find ourselves, as disabled people, in these materials. The exceptions tend to show people with disabilities as sexual victims.

Getting up the nerve to buy erotic material can be hard. It may be easier to go into a more mainstream bookstore than a sex store (they are also more likely to be accessible), but then going up to the cashier with erotica may feel embarrassing. Sex stores may also know more about the titles they carry. Remember that salespeople don't tend to look at what people are buying anyway, and are very unlikely to comment on your purchase, unless it is a book they have read and enjoyed. The best thing to do is rehearse the whole thing in your mind first. Imagine picking out the book, going to the check-out looking cool, handing over your books (you don't have to buy a bunch of books you don't want to cover up the sole erotic one), paying, and leaving with a big smile on your face.

Videos

In the same way that books can fuel a fantasy life, video porn can also add to your sex life, whether by yourself or with a partner. We refer to this material as *video porn* as opposed to visual pornography because porn on video (while primarily visual) also has an audio track, and people who can't see the visuals on screen may still want to rent or buy porn on video. Many people find pornography problematic from a political point of view or moral standpoint. It is often sexist, sometimes racist, and always disability-phobic. The few films that feature people with visible disabilities use nondisabled actors, and the character is always a woman who uses a wheelchair and who is pathetic and horny. They never show her having sex in her wheelchair, but instead it always happens in a dream sequence where, of course, she can walk. Beyond this, the majority of porn is uninspired, lacking imagination, and made for the least amount of money possible. So why are we even writing about it? For many people, despite all this, video porn is still a big turn-on. We want to suggest that even bad porn can be good for some things. Porn is something a lot of us are embarrassed to talk about, but it's a billion-dollar-a-year industry—and many people do rent adult movies. Also, you will find exceptions to the norm: films that are well made, feature good actors, depict believable situations, and show hot sex. And often even in a bad film there will be one scene, one performer, maybe even one fantasy that gets us hot. You need to know how to take what you want from it without expecting too much, employing your sense of humor regularly.

When I suggest that we rent some porn, she acts like I'm some kind of a pervert. Once she went along with it and then she made really stupid comments the whole time, about how unrealistic it was and how ugly the sheets on the bed were. But if I watch it alone I feel like a perv.

Most porn I've seen is terrible! It always seems unbelievable and sometimes makes me embarrassed. But I admit that it still turns me on. Once I suggested to a girlfriend that we watch a movie and I was totally surprised that she had seen lots of porn and was much more comfortable than I was with it.

If you're in a relationship and only one of you likes to watch porn, this can sometimes lead to tension. What seems important is that you find a balance of not putting down each other's sexual desires yet still respecting each other's needs. Your liking to watch porn doesn't make you a bad person, nor are you a prude if you have no interest in porn at all. If you want to try it, ideally you can come up with some rules that will get both of you what you need. It may be that the porn-watching one of you agrees to only watch when your partner isn't there. Of course you can try different kinds of porn and see if there's one you both like.

When choosing a video you should consider what sort of sex you want to see. Films are generally divided into heterosexual (which always include at least one scene between two women, but never a scene between two guys), gay, lesbian, bisexual, and "other." It is a commonly held belief that people only watch porn that fits with their identity ("I'm lesbian so the only porn I would like is lesbian porn"), but in fact one of the interesting things about reading or watch pornography is that it allows us to enjoy watching or imagining something that we don't want to do, or to explore other aspects of our desire safely, without involving anyone else. Lots of straight *and* queer women rent (and love) gay male porn, for example.

You should consider the level of sexual explicitness you want. Everything is available, from films that show no penetration at all to very graphic, raunchy porn that is mostly close-up shots of genitals. If you haven't watched any visual pornography before and you are unsure about your comfort level, you may want to start with less explicit and see how you feel.

Another consideration is plot or no plot. Several directors (most notably people like Andrew Blake and Cameron Grant) use almost no plot at all; rather, their films are just a series of sex scenes put to music with little or no dialogue. Other directors (such as Paul Thomas and Candida Royalle) rely heavily on dialogue and plot. These directors focus more on the interaction between characters, and their characters actually have conversations before they start having sex.

You may also want to consider production values. Most porn is made very cheaply, and it shows. But several companies are producing high-end productions with proper lighting, sound, costumes, and sets.

We recommend you rent porn rather than buy it. Videos are usually expensive, and if you don't know what you like you will probably end up with a few duds before hitting the jackpot, and those duds can cost you.

Adapting Toys

Toys are imperfect, and the best approach to take is that you can make them your own, sometimes by the things you do with them, sometimes by the things you do to them. It's impossible to address every issue people will have about using toys, but below are some guidelines that will get you brainstorming. We'll break this section down by issue rather than by type of toy. The obstacles often overlap. If you have a hard time holding a toy because of a mobility impairment, fatigue may also play a role. Shopping for sex toys when you have a disability usually means having to educate the person helping you in the store (or online). A few years back we did a survey of some of the bigger online retailers to check out their politics and knowledge around disability. We found most stores are very happy to help, enjoy the learning experience, and don't give off a lot of attitude. Before you begin it helps to know what you want to do with your sex toy and any potential obstacles to using it.

Mobility and Motor Control

Having reduced mobility or less motor control of your hands or arms doesn't mean you can't play with sex toys. To start, consider any needs you have in terms of holding sex toys. What do you want to do with the toy? What movement do you have that you can use to manipulate a toy? Where would you want the toy to touch, and can you reach there? If you are thinking about using a vibrator, can you also press it against your body in addition to holding it? If you're interested in a dildo, can you manipulate a toy for penetration? Remember, even if the answer is no to many of these questions, solutions can always be found. Here are a few basic ones.

Some vibrators can be worn on the body so that you don't need to hold them in place—they either go around the waist and sit in front of the clitoris, or they go around the penis and stimulate the penis and scrotum.

There is also a new line of "remote control" sex toys that can be placed near the part of your body that you want to play with and then turned on from a remote switch. These are expensive, but they are very adaptable sex toys. While you may need to get help getting the toys on, and turning them on, many of them will stay on your body, so that you can still play alone if you want. Pillows are also helpful for positioning to play with a toy.

If you can hold a toy and press it against your body but you tend to drop things as a result of spasms, try a vibrator that you can fit on your hand (there's even one so small it fits just on the finger). This type will save you from having to keep getting someone else to pick up that damn vibrator buzzing away on the floor. One company in particular, called Finger Fitting Products, has made a vibrator called the Fukuoku (pronounced *foo-koo-o-koo*). This is a lightweight but surprisingly powerful vibrator that fits on a finger. This is particularly useful if you drop things a lot, as you don't have to keep picking it up. This company has also developed a waterproof vibrating glove that works much the same way and offers the same lightweight vibration.

For some people reach will be an issue. They can try toys that are lightweight but have long flexible shafts that help with reaching areas.

Other folks may also be able to incorporate whatever assistive devices they use for reaching, with a sex toy.

With dildos, using harnesses greatly reduces the amount of movement required. Many people use a harness to affix a dildo to a bed or chair and can then play with the dildo without having to hold it. This takes some practice to get the dildo into a spot you can access comfortably. You can also buy dildos that have suction cups on the base. Usually these are not strong enough to hold the dildo to a wall, but they will keep it grounded on the floor (or a chair) and keep it erect. Another trick with dildos is to buy a much longer dildo than you need. First this helps with grip. Some toys for penetration are so small that once you've got a good grip on the toy you're left with only a few inches to play with. If you need to get a really firm grasp on a toy, it's better to buy something much longer than you would actually use. Another benefit of longer toys is that you can hold a long dildo between your knees to play with a partner.

Handles and switches on sex toys are terrible, and you may need to get a handle built up, or a switch adapted. Finding a friendly occupational therapist is a good place to start. They may be put off by your request, but they may also appreciate the challenge. Going in with a good idea of what you need may help the occupational therapist get over their possible embarrassment. Of course, they may have a huge sex toy collection at home and might be thrilled that they are finally getting to work with something other than cones! If you don't have a place where you use services regularly, we suggest starting with your local center for independent living. Ask them about local adaptive technology programs. If you're still stuck you can approach the sex toy stores listed in the Sexuality: Products section of chapter 14, as some of them may be willing to ask around for you.

Fatigue

I'm looking into "tired top toys"… and have had to experiment with different positions and techniques to minimize the pain and injuries. As a top I can use lighter weight items (tired top toys)…like

a lightweight flogger instead of a heavy whip. I can alternate arms,
so my shoulders don't get too tired.

Low energy and getting tired out can be as great an obstacle as mobility limitations for many people. Timing sex play for times of greater energy or around medications can be a good idea. When thinking about toys, fatigue becomes an issue mostly in the weight of a toy, and the way you might have to hold it. Get something that you can easily put down if you need a break. You can always find lightweight versions of vibrators, dildos, and other toys.

If you are looking for strong vibration but know you won't be able to hold a heavy electric vibrator long enough, you can use some pillows to hold a wand vibrator against you, or to prop yourself into a position that allows you to lean into a vibrator. You may need some help setting this up, but if you have controls that allow you to turn the toy on and off, you can play in private. You can also have a wand type vibrator placed between your legs if you are sitting up. Because the vibrator stimulates a large area, even if it isn't resting exactly where you're most sensitive, the vibration is often more than enough for a good time. These vibrators are great for lying beside or placing between you and a partner. One safety concern is that if the motor is completely covered (by, say, a pillow), the vibrator could overheat and burn either the bedding or you. You need to make sure you won't roll over onto the toy, or if you will that you have someone around who can help.

If you're considering a vibrator or anything else with a motor in it, be aware that if you accidentally fall asleep with a vibrator on you or in you, it can pose a serious burn risk.

Decreased Sensation

A great advantage of sex toys is that they can help you explore sensations on all parts of your body. Don't assume that if one part of your body feels a certain way, everywhere else in that general area will feel the same way. The body is full of erogenous zones, and when sensation is lost in one area, you can (and most people do) shift your erotic focus to other parts. There is variation in how sensation is experienced, but having reduced sensitivity need not mean reduced sexual response. In areas of reduced sensation, toys that produce a light touch won't be very useful, while a vibrator can provide needed strength and stimulation. Many people explore sensation toys like paddles, whips, and floggers, which provide a more substantial sensation. Stay aware of the area you are stimulating—for with decreased sensation it is easier to injure yourself with excessive pressure or rubbing without feeling it.

Increased Sensation

People with hypersensitivity find vibrators to be very unpleasant. They simply provide too much stimulation. Remember that sex toys are just toys, and are a matter of taste and preference. With hypersensitivity it is best to get a toy whose movements you control. For example the nonvibrating insertion toys for men can provide intense stimulation merely from having them around the penis. Women can use other toys, usually called *clitoral stimulators,* that are textured pieces of rubber made to be rubbed up against and provide a much milder clitoral stimulation. Homemade toys can be tailored to provide precisely the amount of stimulation you need. Paintbrushes are ideal sex toys as they come in different shapes, sizes, and textures; are easy to use; can be held in a hand, mouth, or foot; are inexpensive; and are easy to clean.

Privacy

Another consideration in adapting toys is the kind of privacy you have when using a toy. This will depend in part on whether you are using a toy with a partner or by yourself, and if you are using a toy with a partner what they can do with it.

Two major considerations when choosing a toy that will be accessible to you is the noise and the cleaning of the toy. Both wand style electric vibrators and hard plastic battery-powered vibrators can be very loud. This could be an issue if you are living with people and you don't want them knowing exactly what you are doing. You might be able to use other sounds, like music, to hide the sound of the vibrator, but if you don't have a lock on your door, someone may still come in to ask you to turn down the music, which would be a surprise for all involved. If you are concerned about noise then choosing a coil type electric vibrator, or a soft rubber vibrator, would be a better bet. If you are shopping in person ask to hear what the toy sounds like when it's turned on, or if you won't be able to hear the difference ask the salesperson for a quieter toy. If you are shopping online, email the store and ask them to recommend some quieter toys.

The second major consideration is the ease with which you can clean the toy. If it's possible, cleaning your own sex toys will obviously give you more privacy. Some toys are easier to clean than others. For example, battery-powered vibrators that are waterproof can be fully immersed in water and cleaned while you are bathing or taking a shower. A nonwaterproof vibrator is more difficult to clean because if you get any water near the cap it will probably damage it. If you can get a condom onto a toy it will extend its life and make cleanup easier. Some cylindrical toys for men are hollow all the way through and very easy to clean just by running a wet cloth through the toy a few times. Others have one end open but the other closed. These are harder to get completely clean as you need to get a cloth in the end of the tube somehow.

Allergies, Multiple-Chemical Sensitivities, Reduced Immune System

Consider any allergies, chemical sensitivities, or reduced immune system issues when choosing a sex toy. Latex allergy is fairly common, and latex is found in most condoms and gloves as well as many dildos, vibrators, and sensation toys. Never assume a toy is latex free. While a lot of mass-manufactured dildos are not made from latex, they are often poured into molds that have come into contact with latex, in factories where latex is being used. People with serious latex allergies need to be careful about this as retail stores will rarely know exactly where a toy came from. The one exception to this is silicone dildos. Most of the silicone manufacturers work only with silicone rubber and thus can guarantee no latex in their products. Apparently some manufacturers do use latex in their molds, so again it's always best to ask.

If you have a latex allergy, there are alternatives for both toys and safer sex gear. There are now three kinds of nonlatex male condoms and one nonlatex female condom being manufactured. All these products are made from polyurethane, and while they come with their own limitations (they cost about $2 per condom) they offer options for people with severe latex allergies. For more specific information on these products see chapter 12 on safer sex. Most of us don't have sex with kiwi fruit, but if you are latex allergic you shouldn't eat them either, as they are in the same family as the trees that make latex.

Lubricants, creams, and oils, as we've noted above, can have many ingredients, some of which may cause an allergic reaction or direct chemical irritation. People who work in sex toy stores don't usually know much about the details of the products they carry. If ingredients aren't listed on a product, and you really want to buy it, you may be able to write to the manufacturer and possibly get a reply. Or if your allergies aren't life threatening, you can try rubbing a small amount of the product onto your inner arm and see if a rash develops over the next few hours.

Unfortunately, more and more toys designed for penetration (whether they vibrate or not) are being made with a scented rubber. Manufacturers are doing this to hide the unpleasant smell of the less expensive rubbers they use. But the scent is sometime strong and can induce a reaction. Again, when buying toys, it's best to ask whether the toy is scented. If the salesperson doesn't know, insist on being able to open the package and smell the toy before you buy it. Also, some people will react to the dyes in toys for penetration. If you don't have a latex allergy the easiest way to deal with all these concerns is to use condoms on all your sex toys.

Anyone who is immunocompromised (immune suppressed, reduced immunity) should be very careful about cleaning sex toys. You may want to consider buying smaller amounts of lube or creams so that they are used up quickly and don't have time to grow germs in them.

Safer Sex with Sex Toys

In chapter 12 you will find a longer discussion of safer sex in general. But for now, the basic facts to know about safer sex with sex toys are much like the basic facts about safer sex itself. Many sexually transmitted infections (STIs) can be carried by sex toys, even those that have been washed with soap and water.

You can get an STI from using a toy used by someone else with an STI, even if it was cleaned in between. If you have an STI you can reinfect yourself with a sex toy. We recommend always using condoms if you are going to share toys with someone else, or if you have an infection you are trying to get rid of. Other bacteria can also live on toys, so it is not safe to use a toy anally and then use it vaginally, unless you use a condom and change the condom in between. Condoms will also increase the life span of less expensive rubber toys. The one exception to these rules is toys made from silicone. Because silicone can be boiled, you can safely use these toys both anally and vaginally, and share them, as long as you boil them in between uses. You need to be realistic about your time for cleaning toys. If boiling your dildo is not going to be convenient, you need to use (and change) condoms when moving a toy from anus to vagina.

Monitoring Your Own Body Responses

Safer sex with toys involves having an awareness of body responses and making sure that sex toys don't cause problems you may not have considered. Sensation toys are a good example. Playing with a flogger or whip may open up a range of body responses you hadn't considered before. If you are unable to tell (or visually check) that your skin is okay (for example, not being broken), being flogged may be risky. Some lubricants and creams will increase the chance of yeast infection and urinary tract infections. Having a way of checking yourself out is an important part of safer sex.

Autonomic dysreflexia (AD) can be triggered by using a vibrator. Knowing about AD and having a plan to address it if it happens is crucial. See chapter 12 for a more detailed explanation and discussion of AD.

Where to Buy Sex Toys

You can select sex toys in stores, by mail order through a great many catalog companies, and on a huge number of sites on the Internet.

Stores

Whenever possible it's best to buy products in person. It is easier to find accessible stores that carry adult books and videos than toys. Most mainstream bookstores have an erotica section, and even the big chains are carrying some pretty smutty titles. While the big video stores usually don't carry porn, many independent video stores have an adult section, and some will be accessible.

Mail Order

There are a few big mail-order companies in the United States that will send you a paper catalog, letting you ponder your choices and then make your purchases through the mail. These companies tend to have a lot of toys and videos, but few books. We recommend only dealing with companies that have active 800 (toll-free) telephone numbers that offer customer service on the phone. Many of these companies will charge for their catalog but offer you the money back toward your first purchase. Before you do place an order the first time, we recommend that you call with a few questions. Judge what their service is like from their responses. Do you feel like they are rushing you off the phone? Does everything they say sound like a sales pitch? If you can't think of anything specific to ask, inquire about their return policy. If something breaks what can you do? Who pays for shipping a broken toy back to the company? As far as we know there aren't any mail-order companies that have TTY/TDD phone lines available. But again, using a relay service and gauging the company's responsiveness can give you some idea about how supportive they are of all their customers. Chapter 14 lists some recommended companies.

Online

The Internet has proven to be a great boon for sex toy shoppers. It is an easy way to compare prices, check out a company's customer service, and get very specific information, all with zero travel (if you have a computer at home) and without spending any money up front. Hundreds of online companies will be happy to sell you sex toys, books, and videos. In the United States there are also websites that let you rent porn (they mail you the videotape or DVD and you mail it back to them). As with the paper catalogs we recommend that you check out a company before making a purchase. First, visit their site and have a good search around. Then email them a question or two. Based on how quickly they respond, and what their response is, you will probably get an idea of the sort of company they are. Only a few sites offer specific information related to disability, but those that don't may still have information and resources if you ask. The Sexuality: Products section of chapter 14 lists the sites we think are the best.

Yoga and Tantric Sex

When most of us think of *yoga,* we imagine a bunch of sweaty people contorting themselves into unbelievable postures. We know that each person in the group is secretly striving to do the posture more perfectly than anyone else. We also usually imagine something that is vaguely spiritual (possibly cultish). Unfortunately, these assumptions are true for many Western yoga practitioners. But the spirit of yoga is much more than postures, and real yoga is never about competition. It is about focus, breathing, relationships, clarity, and the mind.

All current forms of yoga are based on the Yoga Sutras that were compiled by Patanjali more than 2,000 years ago. Patanjali took from the Vedas (a massive group of sacred texts) everything that was said in them about the mind. The second sutra says, "Yoga is the ability to direct the mind exclusively toward an object and sustain that direction without any distractions." Patanjali went farther than this, directing us "beyond the mind" to a deeper, more essential being. He saw the mind as an instrument that is used by the self. The Yoga Sutras are not about postures. Rather, the postures exist to bring our bodies to a point where we can comfortably focus our minds.

Adaptable Yoga

So, what does this have to do with disability, and what does it have to do with sex? One form of yoga is particularly well suited for people with disabilities. Developed by T. Krishnamacharya in the early 1900s, with the tradition carried on by his son T. K. V. Desikachar and grandson Kausthub Desikachar, it focuses on individual teaching tailored for each student. This type of yoga has been referred to as *Viniyoga*, which means "adaptable" in Sanskrit. (See chapter 14 for information on teachers and workshops). Therefore it does not assume that only one posture works for one type of person. Rather, the needs of each student are taken into consideration. The relationship that develops between teacher and student is of central importance. Each individual develops according to what they need and what they can do. Yoga can help us find the strength and clarity we need to deal with our hectic lives.

In this type of yoga, the assumption is that everyone needs adaptations, and a large part of the teacher's job is figuring out those changes for each student.

Just finding a yoga teacher and getting started is an important part of the process. To begin, we must want to have a relationship with the teacher. For those of us who are shy or who have never sought out a relationship with someone else, this is a step that takes courage and that makes us stronger. We learn as we do this that we don't have to wait for relationships to come to us—that we can go out and find them, negotiate what we need, and be part of a team.

In this form of yoga, much of the movement is felt internally as the body stretches and moves with breathing. Although the postures are important in improving flexibility and increasing strength, their main purpose is in drawing the mind's attention to the body and its possibilities. Viniyoga can be practiced by anyone with any disability as long as they have a teacher who is knowledgeable. It can lead to increased clarity of thought, energy, and control of pain. Desikachar stressed the need to move beyond the mind to the heart, bringing yoga firmly into the realm of community and relationships. In addition to this emphasis, Viniyoga has an impact on sexuality as people practicing it gain an increased understanding of their own body and its capabilities. Improved feelings of self-control can lead to increased abilities, to better know what one wants and to act upon this knowledge.

Healing is an aspect of yoga. Healing is all the processes within our bodies that work to make us healthier. Healing is happening all the time, as little scratches disappear, or as our saliva keeps our throats moist. Yoga doesn't cure disease, but it can help the body improve healing, through a complex interaction of a trusting relationship with the teacher, breathing exercises, and postures.

Yoga and Sex

Breathing is central to Viniyoga. Breathing is also central to sex. The state of calm that is induced by a yoga breathing practice that focuses on exhalation can lead to a decrease in anxiety about sexual performance and an openness to the experience. A practice that focuses on inhalation increases energy and awareness. People who experience difficulties during sex, whether related to previous negative experience or related to disability, can learn ways of breathing that will help them overcome obstacles to having enjoyable sex.

Yoga also gives us a strong sense that we change and learn with practice. Just reading about something is usually not enough. Reading this book will not give you a great sex life, but it will give you ideas of things you can practice to improve your sex life. Some of these things are physical—you can practice kissing or practice pleasuring yourself—but you can also practice different attitudes.

Chanting is not a requirement of yoga, but it is a good way to focus the breath and also focus the mind. Chants do not have to be in Sanskrit or English; in fact they do not have to be in any language at all. You can use words or sounds that are meaningful, perhaps connected to your religion, or just meaningless sounds. Chants can be designed to slowly increase the length of exhalation, leading to pain control, relaxation, and a feeling of calm focus, all of which can also enhance sexuality. Or they can be designed to increase the inhalation, which can be energizing.

For many of us, our bodies seem like the enemy some (or all) of the time. Yoga can give us the sense of a body that is a help, not a hindrance. It can bring us a feeling of control. We may like our bodies more after a yoga practice. It may eventually lead us to a place where we are not composed of different parts, such as mind, spirit, and body, but where our feet or our arms or our genitalia are as much a part of "us" as our thoughts. When we reach this state, we don't think about what to add to the shopping list while having sex. We don't even necessarily think about sex, we *are* sex and sexuality, we are sexual beings experiencing something with all parts of ourselves. Yoga helps us merge consciousness and movement in practices that incorporate postures, breathing, thinking, and feeling, which can have a powerful impact on our sexual expression.

Yoga practices give us time for ourselves, time that becomes increasingly free of distracting thoughts. The practices increase the sense of well-being and self-awareness, both things that can also improve our sense of ourselves as sexual beings.

Most important in this interaction of yoga and sex is the principle that openness to the experience is vital to both realms. Openness involves an acknowledgment that we need to know more, and that we don't always act in ways that assure we will get what we want. In sex, openness may lead to recognizing what we don't want and learning to say no, but also to acknowledging needs and learning to say yes, to ourselves and to others.

Tantra

Sex isn't some new thing that was invented in recent history. We all know this, but we tend to imagine that until recent times sex has been mainly about procreation and not about enjoyment. There are different ways of thinking about sex that are radically different from the current North American approach, and some of these have been practiced for a very long time. One of the oldest approaches is Tantra.

One translation of the word *Tantra* is "tools for expansion." Tantra is over 1,500 years old, and like yoga it originated in India. It consists of a set of teachings and practices that are specifically designed to help us feel more, to increase our awareness of our own energy as well as the energy around us. The path that Tantra uses to these ends is the exploration of sexual energy.

Tantric teachings state that by more fully experiencing our own sexual energy and potential, we are bringing ourselves closer to being one with a universal energy or higher power. These teachings are not about adhering to specific rules or beliefs. Even if we aren't interested in taking on the religious, "higher power" aspects of Tantra, we can take what we like and leave the rest.

Many of the teachings are about desire and the experience of sexual energy. Unlike Western approaches to improving your sex life, these teachings do not revolve around external evaluations of what our body looks like, what kind of car we drive or how we wear our hair. Instead the focus is on our tuning in, to evaluate our minds, spirit, and breath. This focus not only makes a refreshing change from the sorts of pressures we all face, it also offers a centuries-old tradition to consider as a replacement for the standards against which we currently measure ourselves.

Like other kinds of yoga, Tantra is taught by many teachers around the world who have their own take on it, influenced by the cultures they grew up in.

The goal of Tantric sex is to allow us to experience more depth and breadth in our sexuality. The goal is not necessarily orgasm, but rather an enriching of the whole sexual experience. The practice of Tantric sex requires a shift away from thinking about the body as the most important part of who we are.

Tantra explores the distinction made between our physical body and what is sometimes called our "energy body," although it aims to integrate the two. It sees our physical body as what keeps us alive, but our energy body as what gives us life. This does not have to be a religious idea, although the closest thing we have in Western thought to the energy body is the soul.

One of the most radical ideas in Tantra is that our energy body is more important than our physical body when it comes to expanding our sexual experience. It is our energy body that can provide us with constantly new and boundless possibilities of sexual feelings. Our energy body is not judged based on nondisabled norms. Tantra does not require a particular kind of physical body, and truly breaks all the mainstream rules about what sex is all about and how to have it.

Tantra distinguishes many different energy systems within us. One of these that you might have read about already is *chakras:* energy centers in the body between the pelvis and the top of the head. In this system of thought, there is the idea that the smooth flow of energy in our bodies can get stuck somewhere in the system, having been blocked from moving freely or depleted for a variety of reasons. Tantric practice works toward keeping energy flowing through our energy centers smoothly and naturally.

Tantra is different from Western ideas about sex in some other important ways. The Western concept of sex is like a story with a clear beginning (sexual excitement), middle (penetration), and end (orgasm). Sex without penetration is often viewed as being "not real" or "merely" foreplay. Sex without orgasm means that someone has failed, either in not attaining it or not providing it in some way for their partner. In Tantric sex the point of sex is not orgasm, the point is to feel. There is no clear-cut beginning, middle, or end. Most of the exercises related to Tantric sex involve slowing things down, trying not to focus on our external body, or orgasm, or anything outside of our experience of the moment.

Tantra moves us away from a medical model of sexuality and sexual response.

Without a focus on orgasm, Tantra's goal becomes increased awareness, leading to greater understanding of ourselves, which eventually leads to enlightenment. There is no pressure to "get over the top." This doesn't mean that orgasm doesn't exist in Tantra, it just isn't the be-all and end-all. The spiritual practice and the good sexual feelings are interrelated, each leading back to and improving the other.

Another key aspect of Tantra is nonattachment. In our culture we are constantly attaching ourselves to things, objects, people, even rigidly held beliefs. Tantra teaches that these attachments keep us closed to many possible experiences, and to experience deeper knowing we need to gently release our grasp on these things. This doesn't mean we have to give up our favorite boots, or stop believing in things that are important to us, but rather giving things up in the moment, examining what is truly essential to us and what we are holding on to out of anxiety, habit, frustration, or self-doubt. A perfect example of an attachment that can get in the way is our culture's attachment to orgasm. By thinking that there is one goal to sex, and keeping our mind on only that goal, we often miss all the beautiful moments along the way, and sometimes find we are unable to reach that goal anyway.

Mitch Tepper, the founder of sexualhealth.com, wrote a wonderful article about Tantric sex and disability. In it he points to research conducted by Beverley Whipple and her colleagues at Rutgers University. Their work clearly documents cases where women who have complete spinal cord injuries had orgasms from fantasy stimulation alone, orgasms that were not connected to genital contractions. This fact flies in the face of medical understanding of sexual response and points to the variety of other ways to experience sexual pleasure that are open to any of us.

Tantra is about essence. To practice Tantra means you are willing to think about life beyond all that which we normally hold near and dear. It means no longer thinking in terms of body/mind/spirit as three separate parts of ourselves, but rather experiencing them as a whole.

Exercises

In his book *The Essential Tantra,* author and teacher Kenneth Ray Stubbs writes about four common psychological obstacles to Tantric practice.

The first is the idea that in sex we are either a spectator or a performer. If our attention is focused on watching what is going on, what our partner is doing, or how our body is looking or responding, we are taken out of an awareness of the moment.

The second is about judgment. We need to begin to actively stop ourselves when we are judging appearances during intimate moments. It's not that any of us can be wholly nonjudgmental, or that we shouldn't have personal tastes. But if we're doing this judgment either with ourselves when we are alone, or with a partner, during a sexual moment, it is likely that we're doing it as a way of keeping ourselves separate from the experience.

The third obstacle is comparing our current experience with past experiences. We all do this to some extent. But when we focus on this, we are unable to experience things in a new way, to see new possibilities.

The last obstacle Stubbs writes about is having specific expectations of the future. Tantra is about the journey, not the destination. Having our mind fixed on a final goal means we can't focus our energy on what it's like on the path to get there.

Tantra is about receptivity, relaxation, staying in the present and awareness. The breathing techniques and awareness exercises in chapter 3 are essentially yoga and Tantric exercises. If you skipped them before, you may want to go back and give them a try now. As you use your breathing to focus on parts of your body, try to be aware of the ways that your feelings change as you focus your awareness on a particular part of your body. As you are breathing and concentrating on your ears, for example, pay attention to physical feelings, like sensations of heat or cold, vibration, lightness or heaviness, as well as emotions that ebb and flow.

1. Self-Massage

Tantric self-massage involves putting pressure on a point and releasing. If you can do this, pick a part of your body you can apply pressure to. You don't need to do any special breathing with this exercise, but be aware of your breath as you concentrate on the spot on your body you are pressing on. Feel the air passing over the area. Experience the difference between no pressure, then pressure, then release of pressure. If you can't apply physical pressure, use your mind and imagination to concentrate on a point, then release. Imagine the air passing over that point. Do you experience that point differently when you are concentrating on it as opposed to when you aren't focusing? These may seem like simple exercises and in fact they are, but they are good for slowly changing our awareness of our bodies. Be aware of your thoughts as you do the above exercise. If you find yourself losing focus, thinking about other things you need to get done, stop and try to let those thoughts drift out of your mind and shift your focus back to the experience of pressure, no pressure, release of pressure.

2. Separating Orgasm and Ejaculation for Men

In chapter 3 we talked about the fact that orgasm and ejaculation are two separate events in men and women. This is something many men are unaware of if they usually experience both orgasm and ejaculation simultaneously. A great exercise to increase your awareness, which also helps men delay ejaculation, is learning the difference between the two events. This exercise only applies to men who regularly ejaculate and experience orgasm. If you don't usually do one or the other, you probably already know that they are different.

Start by pleasuring yourself in whatever way you like to best, but while you are doing this use the breathing techniques described in chapter 3.

The first couple of times you do this, don't try too hard to focus on a goal, just try to pay attention to what happens to your body as you get more aroused and nearer to orgasm. The reason most men don't realize there is a difference between ejaculation and orgasm is that the signs in the body are very subtle. In most men's sexual response they reach what's called the "point of no return." This refers to the physical state where they are so aroused that they are going to ejaculate, and nothing will prevent that. The goal of this exercise is to recognize that point, and slow yourself down so that you don't go over that point. Begin by paying attention to how your body moves as you masturbate. Do your hips or legs move more, or do they move less, as you get nearer to climax? If you feel tension or stress related to spasms, does that change as you come closer to climax? How does your breathing alter? Some men feel a slight tingling at the base of their penis just before orgasm. You may also notice that the head of your penis gets bigger just before orgasm. Whatever the signs are, spend a few sessions masturbating and paying particular attention to the moments just before you come.

The next step is to stop stimulating yourself as soon as you notice the signs that orgasm is coming. Again, think about it as playing with the "point of no return," getting yourself turned on enough that you're almost there, and then breathing yourself back from it a little bit. At this stage you can try a few things to stop yourself from going over the point. You can physically stop stimulating yourself. You can use your breath to focus the energy flowing in your body; try to imagine it flowing up your body rather than down and out through your penis. You can also flex your PC muscle (if you've forgotten how this works, go back to the exercises in chapter 3) and you can massage your perineum. All of these things will shift your energy slightly and should eventually prevent you from ejaculating. The first couple of times may not work. Don't worry about this. This is one form of practice that you can never do too much of (and even when you don't succeed, it's still a lot of fun!).

As you learn to stop yourself from ejaculating, you may notice that the rise in pleasure, the breathing, the physical sensations, don't go away—because you haven't ejaculated yet. This experience is called, by some, *nonejaculatory orgasms*. The great thing about these kinds of orgasms is that if you have one, you can have many, and you don't need to wait for a period of time between them. These orgasms are not accompanied by the same feelings of release that happen when you ejaculate, but as you learn to have them and as you increase your control of both your breath and the energy these orgasms have in your body, you may discover that they provide even more intense and more long-lasting sensations than the sensation of ejaculation alone.

11

S/M

When I was a teenager, I'd try to twist my body this way and that way so I could make my shorts tight. I'd lift my left knee, which is the only part of me that can move, and drop my thigh on my genitals. The pain turned me on terrifically.

This chapter is an overview of S/M. Whole books have been written on this topic, and, as with other topics in this book, it serves only as an introduction to the subject. If this is something you are thinking of exploring, it would be wise to get more information from some of the resources listed in the Sexuality: S/M and Fetish Resources section of chapter 14.

What Is S/M?

S/M covers a broad variety of activities, from the occasional use of sensation toys to the staging of elaborate fantasies that involve dominance and submission. S/M is an abbreviation of *sadomasochism,* which is described in most dictionaries as a perversion involving getting pleasure from either delivering or receiving pain. This has led people to think that S/M is an illness that involves wanting to really hurt someone, or be truly hurt by someone. In truth, S/M can be a safe, healthy form of sexual expression. Some people are members of an S/M community—it forms a big part of their lives and many of their friends come from the community. For others S/M play may be something they try once and never again, or something done every now and then as part of their larger sexual expression.

While S/M can be defined in many different ways, a basic definition is that it is a form of sexual expression involving a willing exchange of power. S/M play can be physical, involving bondage, restraints, whips, and paddles. Or it can be primarily psychological, using words and imagery to offer submission to someone or actively dominate someone. Many people who have been playing with S/M for a long time also talk about a spiritual aspect to S/M, and say that S/M play can result in self-empowerment and personal growth that carries over to other aspects of their lives.

Because people who practice S/M have to deal with the fact that their sexual expression does not fit the norm, they often find greater acceptance of diversity within their community. S/M requires explicit communication and self-care. Where the norm in non-S/M sex (often called *vanilla sex* by people in the S/M community) is to try to look good and perform sexually, S/M sex is about knowing your own limits and boundaries and respecting them above all else.

S/M does not assume that people magically know what their partners want sexually. Communication is key to S/M. The boundaries and the general framework of everything that will happen is discussed beforehand. Sometimes this will be intricately planned out (to the point of the bottom telling the top in advance exactly how to touch them, where, in what order, what to wear, what words to say, and what looks to give). People who are into S/M don't believe that sex must be a spontaneous, psychic event that "just happens." Far from it, they believe that magic and spontaneous emotion can arise from the feeling of being fully in control and empowered by a sexual experience. Once learned, the negotiation skills required for this are transferable to other aspects of life.

Unfortunately, despite their experience as outsiders, people in the S/M community remain relatively ignorant of disability issues, and are particularly ignorant of issues for people living with psychiatric disabilities and psychiatric labels. The most obvious example of this is the mantra of the S/M community: "safe, sane, consensual." These terms refer to the most basic requirements people who practice S/M demand from their encounters. We don't have a problem with the terms "safe" and "consensual" and will get back to these soon.

The term "sane," however, is problematic for us. We imagine the S/M community has taken up this term to fight against the stereotypes of S/M as something that is "sick" or "deranged." But by using the term "sane" they are marginalizing anyone who has a psychiatric illness. If the idea of "sane" play really refers to people being aware of the risks involved in S/M and that the choice to engage in this play is well thought out, perhaps another term could be used. If the S/M community denies access to people with disabilities, people may choose to hide their disabilities, which can result in unsafe play for everyone involved.

The S/M community can be inaccessible in other ways too. Groups may not be welcoming to anyone with a visible disability, or may host events in places that can't be easily reached.

> I find the leather community here to be extremely discriminatory against people with disabilities in general, and to me in particular. Every time I mention how something isn't accessible, I get massively flamed for it by leaders in the community who don't like to hear anything that might make them "look bad." I found out I was a token crip when I won the state leather title...I ran on a platform

of helping make the community accessible to all of us…but every time I tried to do that, the committee that owned the title would tell me how I was their PR person and my job was to make the community look good (and not say anything negative). Apparently, they thought it made them look good that they would allow a disabled titleholder…but only if I was a polite little crip who told them how great a job they were doing. I finally resigned my title when I realized I could not be an activist and a titleholder at the same time.

I am bisexual, nonmonogamous, BDSM switch. I have found a few disabled players in the BDSM community, though not many. It is hard to be alone. I have found great acceptance of my disability in the BDSM scene, though not too many of the dungeons or play spaces are wheelchair accessible.

I can't speak for other parts of the country but the BDSM community in NYC has a really bad attitude toward disabled people. A friend of mine was refused an opportunity to participate in a major Pride event because of blindness. They claimed their insurance wouldn't cover the involvement because of the disability. Accessibility at most venues is nonexistent and the people in charge are downright arrogant and disrespectful when asked about providing such things.

At the same time, others find support and acceptance in S/M communities.

I have learned a lot from my leather friends. Many of them were able to accept me and all my baggage even when I wasn't. It took me a while to get used to the idea that there were people who were proud to be freaks, I don't think I really trusted them at first, but once I did, and got to know and trust some of them, it's been very liberating. I still have a hard time finding people to play with sometimes, but I wouldn't trade the experiences I've had for anything.

Of course, you don't have to be part of the community to participate in S/M play. Many people integrate aspects of S/M into their sex life without ever considering it to be a lifestyle or anything other than a private activity. Even then, people with disabilities may be faced with stereotypes that hinder this. People may feel that a person with a disability cannot be a top, or that they shouldn't want to be a bottom.

I find it extremely difficult. Even people I am paying don't want to do S/M with me. Getting vanilla sex, even for money, is difficult. The only period of my life was when I had a paid master. I was paying him, however he was calling the shots. I had to end that relationship, as the last time he was here he was doing some sort of drug. Even if you don't have a disability, you must have trust in your master. I am a very vulnerable person and must be very careful. I haven't found anyone to replace him.

I also find that the belief that a disabled person is "weak" or "helpless" keeps a lot of people from taking me seriously as a Top/Domme. A lot of people equate physical strength with being a Domme...even though Domming is so much more in the head than in the body. I was lucky...my mentor was disabled long before I thought I was...and she was an incredible Domme. She was known as a Domme's Domme (and was the only person who could ever get me to say, "Yes, Ma'am" to anything).

The "safe" part of the three basic concepts in S/M means that whatever a person wants to do, from tying someone to a bedpost to piercing someone's skin with a series of temporary piercing needles, they need to know the safe way to go about it. They need to have whatever equipment is necessary to play safe and they should have plans in case something goes wrong. They must be able to provide support for whatever might be needed by their play partner(s) once they are done (which is referred to as *aftercare*).

S/M play is, and must be, consensual. All parties involved are aware of what is going to take place, have agreed to be there and to engage in the play. Anyone has the right to withdraw their consent at any time. This basic concept is one of the empowering aspects of S/M play, because it means that every time we play we acknowledge the power to choose.

S/M play may involve other kinds of sex (including penetration) but doesn't have to. It is up to the individuals involved to decide.

Many people consider S/M almost like theater. People take on roles and personae and it can have a cathartic effect. When we push our limits, emotions come to the surface, and—like Tantric yoga described in chapter 10—this can lead to self-understanding and feelings of self-empowerment.

Basic Terms in S/M Play

Anyone can try S/M without knowing any terms. As long as you figure out what is safe, what you feel comfortable with, and have planned for safety, you don't need a special vocabulary. But it's a good idea to know a number of terms used by people who are seriously into S/M.

The *top* or dominant is the person doing things to the submissive or *bottom*. A session of S/M play is called a *scene*. Because power is not a clearly defined entity, and exchanging power from one person to another happens in subtle ways, the definitions of tops and bottoms can change from person to person, and scene to scene. Some people identify only as a top or as a bottom. In all their play they like to just be dominant, or just be submissive. Many other people will switch back and forth, generally preferring one role over the other. We believe that dominance and submission are aspects of all of us.

One of the most misunderstood aspects of S/M is who controls the scene. People who know little about S/M assume it's the top that controls things. But this isn't the case. The bottom really runs the show. They are the ones who set the limits about what they will do, won't do, how they want to be spoken to, touched, and treated after the scene is finished. It is the top's responsibility to take care of the bottom, while both parties participate in the illusion that the top is in control.

BDSM is another common term. The B and D stand for *bondage and discipline,* which are two popular aspects of S/M play.

Safewords are a crucial part of S/M play. Safewords are signals that the bottom uses to indicate that they want the scene to stop immediately. They don't have to be spoken words but can be signs or gestures. Safewords are one way consent is communicated. Before any kind of S/M play begins it is important to establish a safeword. The idea behind safewords is that we not only need to be aware of our limits and learn when we've reached them, we also need to recognize the feeling of being *about* to reach them. It's okay to stop sex at any time and ask for what you need, without its being interpreted as rejection of either your partner or what you're doing at the time.

Typically people will have more than one safeword to indicate what they want exactly. So someone might use the word *yellow* to indicate that they need things to slow down a bit, but not stop entirely. The word *red* could indicate that something is wrong and the scene needs to end right away. Of course it is important that you come up with safewords that you will be able to use at all times. Usually people will invoke their safeword when they are distressed or fatigued or otherwise off. Because those situations may exacerbate communication problems for some people, having a couple ways of communicating is a good idea.

Sometimes when I'm in the middle of a scene I have difficulty finding the safeword to tell my partner to stop. Especially if I'm feeling distressed. I use my good hand to slap on the bed a couple of times to let them know that the scene should stop.

I'm very particular about safewords because my energy can go quickly and I can go from being right there to being out of it in seconds. Everyone I play with knows what extreme fatigue looks like on me. Also, if I'm worried about either forgetting a safeword or being too out of it to use it, I will also use a rubber ball in my hand. When I drop the ball my partner knows to stop what's going on and check in with me. I haven't dropped the ball yet, but it's good to have it there.

When we explore with S/M, the intensity of the play can add to any difficulty in using regular communication that we have. Some disabilities make "word search" difficult, so we can't find the word we want to say. Sometimes we know what word we want to use but can't get it out. In S/M, communication is crucial, and it is important to figure out several ways to communicate before you start to play. So if you usually rely on verbal communication, you may want to come up with some simple hand signals to use for when you're too exhausted (or excited) to say something verbally. If you rely on sign language or other gestures in conjunction with a communications device, maybe you can also use a particular look to communicate something, or a body movement that is easy for you to do at all times. A bell within easy reach, on a string that can be held or strapped to the hand, can be rung as a safeword. A ball or other small object can be dropped or thrown on the floor as a signal.

Another safety issue is that this kind of sex play can be much more psychological than a lot of other kinds of sex, and we need to be more aware of triggers and self-care issues than when we are talking about asking someone out on a date, or kissing. If someone with post-traumatic stress disorder (PTSD) wants to try S/M, their partner must be able to tell if there are warning signs (things they might say, ways they look, sounds they might make) that they are having a flashback or are otherwise distressed.

> I don't play if I am not feeling stable at the time. I work on shielding, and I refuse to do things that I know are triggers. As a Domme, that is pretty easy to do...I have also played with several subs with dissociative identity disorder and PTSD. What I do is to really know the person before playing...what triggers her flashbacks, what helps calm her...where to explore and where to leave alone, etc. Sometimes I do have to stop a scene...I watch for clues and have a good sense of when to stop and when to work through the trigger by continuing slowly and carefully...communication is the key. If I know the sub has PTSD, I am watching for signs of a trigger/flashback. I treat that as a safeword and stop play to deal with

the trigger and help her through the flashback. So, even if the sub doesn't know about the trigger, it's important to tell the Domme that she has PTSD, what signs to look for that she is beginning to be triggered, and what kinds of things help in dealing with flashbacks. It helps that I also have PTSD and therefore have some personal experience in dealing with flashbacks, but that's not required. What is required is careful attention, communication, and lots of aftercare.

A Note About Pain

Most people think of pain and S/M as being the same thing. Because of this, some people involved in S/M don't use the word *pain,* but instead talk about "producing sensations." They also say that pain experienced in S/M play is different because it is chosen. S/M is not about inflicting pain in an aggressive or angry way, or about receiving pain and having to endure it. Pain that you don't agree to, or that happens to you without planning (like having a bad spasm, or chronic back pain, or falling down and hitting your head), is a sensation you don't want, you didn't ask for, and you wish would go away.

Consensual pain is something you do ask for. When you ask someone to spank you, it is a completely different experience than when a doctor sticks you with a needle. You might describe what you feel as pain, or you might experience it as a tingle or a heightened sensation.

Many of us live with pain, inflicted on us by our bodies, our doctors, our illnesses. S/M can be a way to change our relationship to the pain we experience in our daily lives.

One man who did a lot of thinking, talking, and writing about this was Bob Flanagan (see sidebar). When he died he was one of the oldest living people with cystic fibrosis. Bob credited his long life to his involvement with S/M play. He believed that by causing pain to himself, he developed a different relationship to pain. It wasn't that he never again felt pain, or got frustrated, or scared, or despairing. But he believed that taking time out to make other kinds of pain fun, as well as learning that

BOB FLANAGAN

Writer, educator, and performance artist Bob Flanagan did much of his life's work in finding links between his experience of living with cystic fibrosis and the masochism that he saw as being at the center of his sexuality. He was an extreme masochist and spent many years in a master–slave relationship with his partner, Sheree Rose. Flanagan's life and death has been chronicled in an excellent documentary called *Sick: The Life and Death of Bob Flanagan*. He identified as a person with a disability and as a person in the S/M community, contributing to both communities throughout his life and finding both influences equally powerful in his artistic work. He drew a parallel in his own life between his disability and his sexual identities. He once wrote, "I was forced to be in the medical world, so I turned that into something I could have control over instead of something that was controlling me."

Having to spend a lot of time in profound pain both in hospital and at home, Flanagan learned early on that masturbating was one of the few things that would make the pain subside, at least a little. He also noted that when he was sick and in pain he got more attention. On some level, he began to equate pain with love, and thus began his journey of personal masochism. One of his works was a toy chest that was decorated with pictures from medical and S/M sources (a doctor with gloved hands and a face mask, a pair of handcuffs, a little whip). He filled the chest with children's toys that all have double meanings. On the lid he inscribed the following text:

"Mine is the bittersweet tale of a sick little boy who found solace in his penis at a time when all else conspired to snuff him out, or, at the very least, fill his miserably short life span with more than its share of pain, discomfort and humiliation. The penis seemed to thrive on whatever shit the rest of the body was subjected to and rose to the occasion of each onslaught, soaking it up like a sponge, or, to be more succinct, the corpus spongiosum became full of itself and my stupid prick danced in the spotlight of sickness and suffering. That first swat on the ass from the obstetrician's skilled hands not only started my diseased lungs sputtering to life, but it also sent a shock wave through my sphincter, up my tiny rectum, and straight into the shaft of my shiny new penis, which ever since then has had this crazy idea in its head that pain and he could control many sorts of painful experiences, gave him the energy and enthusiasm to endure a very difficult disease. It was also empowering for him to take something that seemed to be so much in the hands of others (doctors, caregivers, family) and make it his own by asserting control over the outcome.

Kinds of S/M Play

S/M play can take many forms. While a lot of people consider it something marginal or strange, in reality most of us incorporate some aspects of S/M play into our sex lives. If you've had a fantasy about being the head of a large corporation and seducing your secretary, or get turned on by the idea of being ravished by some sexy stranger, you're having S/M fantasies. If you've ever tied up a lover with scarves or smacked your partner's ass with your hand, you've had some kind of S/M sex. S/M has become somewhat trendy over the past couple of years (this trend began with Madonna's *Sex* book, which contained many S/M images). This has also meant that S/M has come to be associated with having plenty of money (for all those shiny cat suits) and somehow being a very experienced or very serious "player." In fact, because S/M is all about the willing exchange of power, and we all have some power to exchange, you don't need anything other than your desire and a creative, open mind to start exploring S/M play.

Sensory Control

S/M play helps us explore our senses through *restriction* and *addition*. We can restrict our senses by covering our eyes with a blindfold, our ears with headphones, or various parts of the body with clothing. You can also add sensations or change a familiar sensation. If your partner relies on sight, having them blindfolded and then adding sensation can take them to a heightened state of awareness. Many people respond to sensory control more mentally than physically. Losing a sense completely (but knowing it can be returned at a moment's notice) can be unsettling and a bit scary, but it allows you to tune into other things going on both in your body and in the room around you.

I like to make my boyfriend put a blindfold on and have a bag of different toys I can use to touch him with. I'll use my reacher, a rubber glove, a toothbrush. Each time I change it and he never knows what's next. Depending on how I do it I can make him cackle with excitement about what's next, or be completely afraid.

Fantasy Role-Playing

Giving yourself permission to construct fantasy roles can be freeing, allowing you to put your usual self and responses aside and act in ways that might seem unlike "you." Role-playing can also be gender play (discussed in chapter 6), and allows you to explore the parts of you that are different from the gender you identify with in your daily life.

Fantasies involving discipline are probably the most common in S/M play. Many scenes will revolve around the bottom's being required to do something, and when they are unable to do it the top inflicts some sort of discipline, from mild to severe. Discipline may take the form of physical touching such as slapping, spanking, whipping, or tickling. Some people also play with verbal communication, where the discipline is yelling, whispered threats, or humiliation. With experience, discipline can be in the form of merely a look or a clucking of the tongue that indicates the greater punishment to come.

Many scenes involve fantasy roles. Sometimes these are very elaborate (say, an elevator repairperson working at Wal-Mart who has always dreamed of moving up in the company) and sometimes they are as basic as dominant and submissive, master and slave.

Restrictions on Movement

Also called *bondage*, restricting a partner's ability to move in any way can be a powerful part of a scene. Whether you're tied to a bed, your hands are bound with fleece restraints, or you are suspended from the ceiling, bondage can be an exciting way to explore S/M. It may be the thrill of feeling as if your bottom is at your mercy. It may be the excitement of thinking of all the things you can do while they are restrained.

For bottoms, being able to control the kind of restraint and how long it will last and then to let go and allow yourself to be completely "helpless" can be both a turn-on and very freeing.

When using bondage the bottom is particularly vulnerable, as people cannot usually get out of restraints without assistance. For this reason you should always have firm trust and communication established before including bondage in your play.

Bondage doesn't require any special equipment—it can be all psychological. It is bondage when you tell someone they can't move, or when they *can* move. When we restrict movement, our sensations may be heightened. Even small movements may then be noticed more, or experienced differently. We may also sense the bound part of our body differently once it is released.

Restricted movement that we choose is very different from restricted movement that is not chosen. When we talk about S/M in workshops we've done, some people (usually nondisabled people who have not tried S/M play) question why someone who experiences paralysis would ever want to further restrict how they get around. In our experience, many people who have limited mobility and engage in S/M describe a sense of power they get from being in control of such restrictions. The bottom is in complete control. Choosing to be restrained, and getting sexual pleasure from it, and then being able to choose exactly when the restraints come off, can not only offer an incredible feeling of empowerment but provide an opportunity to change the way we experience the idea of restraint.

Flagellation

Any kind of percussive hitting of someone goes by the general term *flagellation*. Spanking with an open hand or hair brush, whipping with shoe laces or a leather flogger (called *flogging*), using a rattan cane on someone's bare bottom (called *caning*)—all are types of flagellation. Because flagellation has ties to religious traditions, this activity holds a great deal of mystique and power for some, and is often considered offensive by those who have never tried it.

When I ask for a series of slaps or several lashes with a whip, I feel excited and afraid. I think, "How hard will this be?" "How will I feel?" But the fear is like people have described being on a roller coaster. My heart pounds, my breathing gets fast, but it's play fear. I can get really scared about what is coming next, but I know nothing bad is going to happen to me.

Endorphins are chemicals that are similar to morphine that are made by the body in response to pain. Flagellation can cause an increase of endorphins, leading to a feeling of euphoria. In addition, applying pain to one part of the body distracts the brain from other sources of pain, so flagellation can actually be a form of pain relief.

Being on the giving end of a scene involving flagellation can be a heady experience for anyone who has never felt in control, who has always been "done to" by others. Knowing that you are meting out punishment as you see fit, and that the punishment may take a while, or may be over quickly, are all things that you can control. It can give a sense of power in a safe context. It's also a great opportunity to tease and taunt your bottom, making them wait for the next hit. You can mix up the intensity of the sensations, giving both their mind and body a progressively heavier set of sensations.

Flogging can be done effectively with minimal physical effort. See the Positions for S/M Play section at the end of this chapter for ideas on adapting flogging to your energy and needs.

Self-monitoring and knowing what is safe is important. If you won't be able to know when to stop, either because you can't see what is being done or you can't feel all the effects on your body, your partner must take responsibility for safety and provide you with feedback about how your body is doing.

Psychological Play

While all aspects of S/M play bear a psychological component, for some people a scene may be entirely about the minds of the top and bottom. Psychological bondage, for example, could mean that a bottom is not allowed to move from a position until the top gives permission. It might mean that a bottom is required to make uninterrupted eye contact with the top, again until released from doing so by the top. No actual tying up is required. Like some aspects of Tantric sex discussed in chapter 10, S/M play does not require that your body do any one specific thing. In many cases it doesn't require the body at all.

Verbal Play

Another play possibility is talking. It may be that you have specific words that either drive you around the bend or can be used to frustrate you, or you have words that will take you to the heights of ecstasy. While keeping some form of communication going during a scene is crucial for safety, adding an element of talking can be good. What you say will usually be dictated by the roles you both are playing. You might be the understanding teacher, offering soothing compliments to a student who was picked on in the playground. Or you might be the angry cop, yelling at a driver who went through another red light. If you like to talk, or your partner does, think about what words turn you on, or press your buttons. Sometimes talking about this kind of thing can be embarrassing and feel very revealing. If you don't want to talk about this beforehand, once you've established what you're going to do in a scene, you can write down or type out for your partner the kinds of things you like to hear. This has the added benefit of your partner's being able to surprise you unexpectedly with some of what you've told them about.

Where to Start

The place to begin is desire. Start thinking outside the normal confines of what is sexual and what is sexual behavior. Scan your memory for things that you associate with some sort of sexual excitement (maybe a sexy movie you saw when you were too young to consciously put it together, maybe a teacher or family friend, or a second cousin whom you had a childhood crush on). Remember that there are no taboos in your fantasy life. Let your mind go wherever it wants. You may choose not to use a certain fantasy in an actual sexual encounter, but there's no harm in letting yourself explore it in the privacy of your mind.

Finding Partners

As always, this can be the tricky part. You have many things to consider when looking for a suitable partner.

Online

Some people participate in S/M play only online. Online play can be a good way to get started. It is a safe way to meet people with similar interests and explore your desires without having the risk of a real-life encounter that might be too much.

In his book *S/M 101: A Realistic Introduction,* Jay Wiseman writes that it is best to start by finding someone you are personally compatible with, as opposed to someone with a specific shared interest. Think about the kind of person you can imagine playing with. S/M play is intense and personal, so it usually means that you need to know the person at least a bit before playing with them. If you find someone who shares your interests but with whom you have nothing else in common, it probably won't work out so well, nor last very long.

In chapter 14 we list some of the larger resources for meeting people in the S/M community. The information in chapter 4 about meeting people through ads and online dating websites applies to finding S/M partners as well. The other main place to find partners is in clubs.

S/M Clubs and Fetish Nights

Most major cities have an active S/M club that holds regular parties. These clubs usually have some equipment and have staff who ensure that everything going on is safe and that if people need assistance they get it. Many of these clubs hold a regular "fetish night." They usually impose a dress code on these nights, but that doesn't mean you have to have a $2,000 outfit to get in. It just means you can't wear jeans or regular street clothes. It's a good idea to call ahead and find out what their dress code is, whether they have change rooms there to switch out of your street clothes, and to ask about accessibility. If you try one place and it is inaccessible, be sure to ask them if they know of any groups that hold accessible events and suggest that they start doing so too.

> I went to a fetish party a number of years ago that was in a rela-
> tively accessible location—I only had to go up two stairs instead of
> a flight of them (what I call "pretend accessible"). I really wasn't
> sure what to expect but was pleasantly surprised. There were all
> types and shapes of bodies and it felt quite easy for me to be there.
> I really just wanted to watch for the first time and people were fine
> with that. There were others there too who were just "watching"
> and they would make room for me with my walker so I could get
> close without my being the center of attention. I have been trying
> to find play parties that are accessible and where I can go without
> bringing someone with me who isn't going to be my partner. This
> has not always been easy but at times, getting assistance from
> someone while I'm there has facilitated my connecting with
> current play partners.

Online Clubs and Social Groups

A lot of online discussion groups are S/M themed. Some get very specific. When you find a group you think you might like, just hang back and observe for a bit to find out if it's a safe place to be and to get a sense of how group members interact.

Negotiating a Scene

Once you've found someone you want to play with, you can begin to negotiate the scene. This includes where you want to play, establishing safewords, safety, what you want to do, and aftercare.

S/M is something most people do at home, either theirs or their partner's. This can be an issue for people living in an institutional setting, because you never know who is going to just walk in. S/M clubs usually provide a space where you can play privately, or some people like to be watched and so they play in the club's public spaces.

Dealing with other people's ideas about what is okay for a disabled person, and what isn't, can be a big issue if you chose to try public S/M.

My partner doesn't look disabled and I use a wheelchair. The few times we've played in public (with me as a bottom) she has had people come up to her afterwards and actually say to her they think she's crossing a line. Like somehow because I'm in a wheelchair I can't be a powerful bottom. It's also ridiculous because she is disabled too, they just don't know that. The first time it happened I was so angry I didn't want to go back to that club at all.

I'm a bottom and it's hard for me to find people to top me. I think even the few people who would are worried about what other people will say about them.

Having found the place and established your intent, you also need to agree on your safewords. You should think about this before you meet: Think of words, gestures, or sounds that you will be able to remember when you are excited or scared. Again, if you anticipate communication being an issue, you may want to come up with two different ways to utter your safeword.

Now you can talk about what you want to do. This is a good time to tell the person anything you have learned from previous experience, especially about anything that you don't want them to say or do. Your plan doesn't have to be elaborate. It can be as simple as "I'd like you to spank me." Go into as much detail as you need to get what you want. If you wish to act out a fantasy, then discuss your roles and a plan for how it will go.

Incorporated into this planning will be a discussion of safety issues. This should include any information about your disability that you think is relevant for the scene you are planning. You are not required to disclose your entire medical history, although some partners seem to expect this. If you are on any medication; if you have any communication obstacles, allergies, fatigue issues, or problems related to bruising or bleeding; or if you are not able to monitor your own body responses, then it is important to discuss these with a partner and come up with plans to deal with all safety issues.

Because S/M play can bring up many feelings and memories, it is important to decide what will happen once the scene is over. Do you want your partner to hang around after the scene to debrief, just talk, or do something completely unrelated to the scene? Do you need to be alone for a while, but then want the freedom to call and talk about it? If a scene becomes emotional for you, do you like to be touched or held when you are upset, or do you need space to feel safe?

Positions for S/M Play

As with other sexual activities, there are many possible positions for S/M, most of which can be adapted with pillows, furniture, and imagination.

> When I do play I can't play standing up or bent over. Basically, my back needs to be straight. I have a lot of problems with female tops because so many seem to tie their involvement in the BDSM scene to ego and have a hard time accepting the fact that they can't do whatever they want when they play with me. I don't suffer fools gladly and on several occasions I've verbally skewered several.

> I like to be spanked before we have intercourse, it gets me really excited. I don't have a lot of strength. Sometimes I lie on the bed on my belly but it can be hard to breathe that way. So usually I kneel on the couch with my belly up against the couch back with my arms over the back of the couch. That way I'm supported and not distracted by concentrating on holding myself up or breathing.

If using the position described above, make sure the couch is well padded along the top where the frame is, so that there isn't too much

TIPS FROM A TOP

I can make sure the bottom is bound in a position I can easily reach from a sitting position. Making sure the bottom is lower than I am helps, since I can use gravity to my advantage.

I can use knives, ice, wax, electricity (something I really want to learn more about and collect toys for), clamps, clothes pins, and so on…they take little physical effort for me and have wonderful effects on the bottom. With a blindfold, the possibilities become even more, as the mind will imagine much worse than is actually happening.

If the play becomes sexual, I have to carefully choose my position in order to not get too tired or injure myself…but the options are limitless.

Remember to explore the psychological, not just the physical. The possibilities are even more limitless, as Domming is much more in the mind than the body. Possibilities include all of what I listed above as a top, plus: having the sub do service, getting into her mind, doing role-play, sensation play.

pressure on the skin or on the circulation. You can pad the top with a folded towel or blanket. You can also sit backward or sideways on a kitchen chair.

People who can't kneel can try lying on a bed face down and place a pillow or two under the abdomen and pelvis, leaving the ass up a bit. The feet can be secured together or apart. Or the top can actually lie on their back with the bottom on top of them. The top can reach around to spank or cane the back and sides of the bottom's body.

Some people are comfortable draped over those big balls that physical therapists use.

Some people are more comfortable lying on one side. The legs can be curled up or kept straight, giving access to the ass, thighs, stomach, and back.

Self-care is very important in S/M play, and there is no technique or toy that is good for everyone. As always, foresight and experimentation are your best bet. There are no rules about who is allowed to do what, and there are no "conventions of disability correctness" that must be followed.

Chapter 9 has a section about sensation toys. All sex toys are really sensation toys, but these are the ones that aren't intended to penetrate or be penetrated. They include paddles, whips, floggers, feather boas, ice cubes, fans, and anything else that will produce an interesting feeling. Always familiarize yourself with toys before you use them. Make sure you get the feeling you want and that they don't have dangerous edges. Check out the grip. See what the weight is like and decide whether you can handle it. Certain toys (such as electrical toys and certain kinds of restraints) may remind you of nonconsensual experiences, in an unpleasant way.

Toys that clip on to the body, like clothes pegs, nipple clamps, and many toys made for "cock and ball torture," instead of being swung, like whips and paddles, may be easier to use if strength is an issue, but coordination and hand strength are more important for these. Light toys are easier to swing, such as a crop instead of a flogger.

Restraints should not rub and should be easy to release. "Panic snaps" are available for some restraints and allow for quick release from bondage.

> I used to be an extremely heavy S/M player as a bottom. Before my disease became serious I was able to transmute pain into pleasure. Now because of my disease even light play is rather painful.

> I got home one night and my girlfriend told me to go upstairs and lie on the bed in the dark with no clothes on. I lay there for what seemed like a long time, my ears straining to hear something. Then all of a sudden, there was a loud noise (she told me after that she had dropped a book on the floor) and then she spanked me very softly all over my back and bum and legs. I didn't know where I would feel it next or if she would start spanking me harder. It was very exciting.

Canes and rods of Delrin or Lexan are flexible and light. They can be handled easily and come in a variety of lengths so that they can be used even if you are unable to get very close. A cane can be strapped to a hand or arm for someone who can move their arm but is unable to grip. Feathers can be used to tickle or stroke. Ice cubes can provide a surprising feeling and can be used by most people. If there is difficulty gripping, a Popsicle maker can be used to make larger ice cubes with a handle. Ice should, however, not be used on areas of poor circulation or held by anyone who has Raynaud's syndrome (where the fingers or toes go numb and white when exposed to cold or vibrations).

Melted wax produces an intense, hot sensation but is not hot enough to burn most people's skin. If you are interested in experimenting with hot wax, it's best to use plain white candles, as colored candles tend to melt at a higher temperature and will be more likely to burn.

Rubber gloves worn when spanking will increase the sensation and are often used by people who don't have enough energy to spank as hard as they would like. If latex allergies are a concern, several types of nonrubber gloves are on the market that feel the same and have the same impact (see chapter 12). Metal fingernails (or even banjo picks) can be run along the skin.

Temporary piercing is said to produce an endorphin rush. It is important to make sure that anything you use is very clean. Do not use the same needle on more than one person. Be very careful about the part of the body that is pierced. Piercing should not be done on anyone with a bleeding disorder.

If you are a top and can't move around easily, you can have the bottom do the moving as part of psychological dominance.

At its core, S/M is about exploring our desires, it's about opening ourselves up to more of who we are sexually, and it's about communication. It's unfortunate that in our culture so many negative ideas are attached to S/M. And while it isn't a kind of sexual expression that is for everyone, most of us can probably find a part of our lives where S/M ideas and practices can offer us new possibilities for personal expression.

12

Sexual Health

Most people have heard the term *safer sex* and many people think it is all about condoms. In fact safer sex is about more than preventing sexually transmitted diseases. It includes aspects of mental, emotional, and physical health and safety. Although it includes doing what you can to keep yourself free of disease and unwanted pregnancies, it is also about keeping yourself free from sexual coercion and being damaged by the actions of others.

We use the term *safer sex*, not *safe sex*, because there is risk tied to everything. Nothing in the world is 100 percent safe, and rather than pretending that anyone can be completely free of harm, we prefer the approach where we do what we want or need to do—but take as many precautions as we can to reduce the risk of harm.

It's important to get as much information as you can (knowing that access may be limited and you have the right to act without having all the information available to others) and then make decisions based on assessing the risk. Risk is hard for most of us to really understand, because if you have a negative consequence, you have it 100 percent. And if you don't, it's zero. So, when someone says, "You have a 10 percent risk of X," how can we really get it? At least if we know what the risks are, we can say, "It would be terrible for X to happen and I will avoid it at all costs," or "I don't really want Y to happen, but there is a low risk and a high chance of something good happening. I can make the risk even lower by protecting myself in some way, so I'll do that." Of course, much of the time, we can't tell you what the risk is for any activity. It is hardly ever as clear as "If you jump off a twenty-five-story building you will almost surely die."

Self-Monitoring

Safer sex information often assumes that we have the ability to be aware of our physical and mental state. But this is not always the case. Lack of privacy is one barrier to self-monitoring. If you are never alone with your clothes off, or partly off, how can you look at your penis or vulva? If you have no feeling in the area, you have no sensation of pain or tingling. If someone else puts your tampon in for you, will they notice anything unusual and will they tell you about it? If you have always been protected against risks, how will you know which feelings to trust when you are making decisions that involve risk?

These limitations don't mean that we can't self-monitor, but we do need to be acquainted with our limitations and figure out ways around them. A person who can't see may want to inspect their genitalia with their fingers regularly to feel for new lumps, areas of roughness, or areas that have a different sensation in them. If you can't arrange for privacy, ask for regular appointments with your doctor to check your genital area if you are having sex. Ask an attendant whom you feel comfortable with to hold a magnifying mirror so that you can see your genitals when they are washing you or dealing with tampons.

All kinds of sex can have effects, both positive and negative. We can figure out what these effects are when we can tell that something has changed, physically, emotionally, or mentally. As you read this chapter, consider the ways these effects might make themselves known, and if you need assistance in monitoring these effects, consider how you might get that assistance and from whom.

Sexually Transmitted Infections (STIs or STDs)

Although the common cold, mono, and the flu can all be transmitted during sex, we don't think of them as STIs (sexually transmitted infections, also known as sexually transmitted diseases, or STDs) because it isn't the sexual contact that causes this, just close proximity. Most STIs cause problems in the genitalia, anus, or mouth, although Hepatitis B is considered an STI and infects the liver. There are also things that seem to be related to having penetration but aren't usually passed from one person to another, like yeast and bladder infections in women.

Infections are caused by germs. Some germs are bacteria, which are fairly large (in the microscopic world) and can be killed by antibiotics. Some germs are viruses, which are much smaller and harder to kill, although there are some drugs now that work against certain viruses. Many people who have STI germs in their bodies have no sign of this— no discharge from their penis or vagina, no funny sores. Condoms stop many viruses and bacteria, but if the germ is in an area that isn't protected by the condom, then you can still get the infection.

Chlamydia

The fairly common STI called chlamydia is caused by something called an "obligate intracellular parasite," which means that it has to live inside cells and doesn't kill the cell. But it causes lots of problems, and like gonorrhea can go to other parts of the body. Chlamydia can cause sterility in both men and women. Most women and many men have no symptoms from chlamydia, but when there are symptoms they include discharge, burning with urination, spotting after penetration, painful penetration (in women), and swelling or pain in the testicles. If there is a discharge it may be smelly. If someone is going to get symptoms, they appear in seven to twenty-one days. There are two kinds of tests for chlamydia, both of which require a swab like a Q-tip. It can be treated with one dose of an antibiotic that is taken by mouth.

Gonorrhea

The bacteria that causes gonorrhea can infect both men and women to cause throat, cervical, urethral, and anal infections. About 80 percent of women don't have any symptoms when they have it. Most men with gonorrhea have symptoms, the most common being a pus-like (usually yellow) discharge from the penis or burning when peeing. Women can get a yellow or green discharge from the vagina and may also have burning when they urinate or pain during penetration. The discharge can be smelly, a very different smell from normal discharge. In women, the infection can go to the uterus and fallopian tubes and cause intense pain. If not treated this can lead to infertility or an increased chance of tubal pregnancies, which is dangerous. A tubal pregnancy is when the sperm and egg meet up in the fallopian tube (this part is normal) and then get stuck there instead of moving into the uterus. The tubes are small, and as the embryo grows, the tube can burst. Less commonly, gonorrhea can go to the joints. If someone is going to get symptoms, they start to show up within ten days of contact. Testing for gonorrhea is done by sending a sample that is collected with something like a Q-tip (for men's urethras, a tiny one) to a lab for culture. Gonorrhea is treated with one dose of an antibiotic that is taken by mouth. There should be a repeat test done two weeks later to make sure it is clear. Many people who have gonorrhea have chlamydia at the same time.

Herpes

Herpes is caused by a virus. The worst thing about it is that after it goes away it can come back many times. Symptoms can occur within a few days of being infected, but can take up to twenty days to appear. Herpes shows as one or more painful blisters that can open up to become sores.

At first they may just be red, painful lumps, but then they become filled with fluid and may look shiny. They are somewhere between soft and hard. They usually appear on the vulva or penis, in the pubic hair, or in the anal area, although they can show up in other places. If they are on the vulva or penis there can be severe pain with peeing. When the infection first happens there can be swollen glands in the groin, fever, headache, and fatigue in addition to the rash. Not everyone gets herpes back again after the first time, and you may be less likely to get it again if treated with antiviral drugs. Some people find that their recurrences are triggered by certain foods, heat, or stress. Herpes can sometimes be transmitted to another person even when there is no rash. Condoms are not always protective, as the rash can occur in areas that aren't covered by a condom. Cold sores are also caused by a herpes virus. Although one version of herpes is more common in cold sores, the other more common in genital herpes, you can get genital herpes if someone with a cold sore goes down on you, and they could get cold sores from going down on you if you have genital herpes.

Human Immunodeficiency Virus (HIV)

This virus is transmitted through oral, vaginal, or anal sex, as well as by getting infected blood into you (from sharing needles or from a transfusion) and through breast milk. Blood is now tested for HIV before being used for transfusion. HIV causes AIDS, which is a disease that makes the immune system function poorly so that the person is prone to other infections and some types of cancer. When someone first acquires HIV, they might get an illness a bit like the flu, with fever, headaches, rash, and joint pain. After that, it can be years before symptoms appear. There is no way to tell if someone is HIV infected by looking at them or at their genitalia. HIV is diagnosed with a blood test. Before having the test, you should talk with someone about how you are likely to react to either a positive or a negative test and make plans. For a while, people were recommending using a lubricant (or prelubricated condoms) containing Nonoxynol-9, a spermicide, to prevent HIV transmission. There is no evidence that this actually works, and some women get vulvar or vaginal irritation from this, which might increase the risk of transmission of HIV. Although many treatments for AIDS have been developed, there is no cure. Much of the recent emphasis on safer sex is a result of AIDS.

Human Papilloma Virus (HPV)

At least sixty human papilloma viruses exist. Some cause genital warts, which can be uncomfortable or even painful. They don't always hurt, though, and many women notice they have them when they feel a bump when wiping themselves. It is unlikely that an attendant would notice them unless there were a lot of bumps. The bumps look a bit like tiny cauliflowers. They usually feel quite hard and not smooth. There can be tiny individual ones, or larger clumps. Warts inside the vagina aren't painful. Some types of HPV have been shown to lead to cervical cancer or rectal cancer. Not every woman who gets HPV ends up with cancer. HPV is probably stopped by condoms, but may be in areas that aren't covered by condoms. People can pass the virus along even when they don't have warts, or none are visible. Treatments are available that make warts go away, but they don't kill the virus. Warts are usually diagnosed just by being looked at. Effects of HPV on the cervix are diagnosed by a Pap smear.

Intestinal Parasites

Parasites can be transmitted through analingus or if a sex toy is shared and used anally. They can cause diarrhea and abdominal pain. There are different treatments for different parasites.

Pelvic Inflammatory Disease (PID)

PID occurs in women and is a result of any number of STIs (and occasionally other infections), most commonly gonorrhea and chlamydia. The infection travels upward from the vagina to the uterus, fallopian tubes, and ovaries. PID can cause sterility, tubal pregnancy and chronic pelvic pain. You can get PID more than once, and each time it occurs your chance of becoming infertile increases. Symptoms include vaginal discharge that varies depending on what kind of infection it is, long or painful periods, spotting and pain between periods, lower abdominal pain, fever and chills, nausea and vomiting, and pain during penetration. PID is usually treated with IV (intravenous) antibiotics. It is diagnosed by a doing a combination of procedures such as a pelvic examination, taking a swab for culture, blood tests, and sometimes laparoscopy (looking at the tubes and ovaries with a little camera inserted through a small cut in the belly button).

Pubic Lice (Crabs)

Lice are tiny insects that can cause intense itching in the genital area. They cement their eggs (nits) to the shaft of pubic hairs. Most people start itching about five days after becoming infested. They are spread during sexual contact and from contact with bedding or clothing that is infested.

If you take a close look, you can see little light-colored dots moving around. With a magnifying glass they look like tiny crabs. They live off human blood. Lice are not dangerous, but they are a real nuisance. Many treatments are available from drugstores. You can also try heavily coating the whole area with petroleum jelly and leaving it on for several hours, which smothers the lice. This can be really hard to wash off, so it is a treatment to use only if you are desperate. You must wash all your towels, bedding, and any clothing you have worn since a week before you noticed symptoms. Vacuuming is also a good idea.

Syphilis

These days syphilis is not very common in North America, which is a good thing because it can have many bad effects on many parts of the body and can be fatal. It is diagnosed by a blood test. The most common symptom is a painless bump, but some people get a rash on other parts of their body. It is cured with a penicillin shot. It is transmitted through intercourse and condoms are protective, unless there is a bump (called a chancre) that is not covered by the condom.

Trichomonas

A small parasite causes trichomonas, producing a frothy, smelly dis- charge and causing pain during penetration for women. It can also cause more frequent, burning peeing. Men don't usually get any symptoms. It can take up to a month to get symptoms after being infected. Women with trichomonas have a higher risk of another germ (like gonorrhea) getting into their tubes and causing pelvic inflammatory disease. Within a week to ten days after treatment with a medication taken by mouth, it is resolved. The medication cannot be taken by women who are pregnant and can cause vomiting, especially when combined with alcohol.

Protection from STIs

You can do a number of things to protect yourself from STIs and their effects. The first is to talk to potential sexual partners about STIs. People can lie, but often they are truthful and you can find out if they have had an STI before, when was the last time they had sex with someone, and whether they have been tested for HIV or other STIs. You can ask them questions like Do they use condoms all the time? Are they willing to have nonpenetrative sex to reduce the risk of STIs? If they haven't been tested before, how would they feel about getting tested?

> I remember when I had to be tested for an STD. I was naïve and trusted what my lover had told me about his sexual history. I didn't know very much about how STDs affected men, so I ended up leaving the doctor's office feeling that my partner knew and just didn't care. But when we talked about it I found out that he had no idea that he had also had an STD. We both got treated and were able to resume our sexual relationship, but we're using condoms. I didn't want to take any more chances.

It is clear from the section before this that there are often no signs of an STI and that you can't tell from looking at someone whether they are infected. You also can't be sure you aren't passing something along, particularly if you have been having penetrative sex without a condom. It doesn't hurt to get tested about two weeks after you have had sex with a new partner. You can get tested for HIV anonymously. That means that no record of the test will show up in your medical record. Some people want to have this kind of privacy because they don't want an insurance company to know their HIV status. Others are worried that their medical record might not be confidential. The disadvantage of this kind of testing is that you have to remember some kind of code word to get your results, as they won't be filed under your name. Also, if you are HIV positive, you might want medical personnel in an emergency room to have this information if you can't communicate it to them. Public health departments usually have a list of who does anonymous testing and should be able to tell you which clinics are accessible.

Using a condom for penetrative sex makes sense. People in long-term relationships who trust each other not to have sex outside the relationship often stop using condoms, especially if they don't need them for birth control.

If you aren't going to use a condom for oral sex, then you should try to avoid getting semen in your mouth. This isn't totally protective, as pre-cum can also have germs in it, but it does reduce your risk. Do not brush your teeth right before sex because it can cause little scratches in the gums that might let in viruses. Some people suggest rinsing your mouth with an antibacterial mouthwash afterward, but there is no evidence that this works.

EASY-ON CONDOM

There is a new condom called the EZ-On. This condom is made of nonlatex material and is unique because of the way it can be put on. Each condom comes in a cardboard disk that offers you something more to hold on to while you slide the condom on a penis or dildo. The design is also unique because you can slide the condom on either way (with most condoms there is a wrong way to slide it on and it won't roll down correctly if you don't do it the right way). This condom has two main drawbacks. First, at the time we wrote this it was not available in the United States. It is currently only available in Canada and Europe. Second, the condoms are very expensive (usually $3 each). For more information about this condom you can visit the company's website at www.mayerlabs.com.

How to Use a Condom

Condom use goes against the environmental "reduce, reuse, recycle" idea. We'd like to see people using *more* of them, and they should never be reused.

Putting on a condom can get tricky if both partners have difficulty using their hands. It takes quite a bit of manual dexterity to open a condom packet and put on a condom. In chapter 4 we discussed negotiating with attendants about putting on condoms. After we describe how to put a condom on with your hands, we will describe a way someone can put one on with their mouth.

Condoms should be put on before the erect penis gets near the partner's genitalia. Condoms come individually wrapped, in little plastic or foil packets. They have an expiration date on them and should not be stored in hot places (like a back pocket or wallet).

Open the packet, being careful not to tear the condom with your teeth or fingernails. Pull the condom out, but don't unroll it yet. Make sure the condom is the right way up. This means you can see the rolled-up part, it isn't tucked inside the condom. Squeeze the tip of the condom so there is no air in it (which makes room for semen). Most condoms have a kind of nipple at the end for this, although a few brands don't. If you want you can put a couple of drops of lube inside the condom (this will increase sensitivity). With the tip squeezed, hold the condom against the top of the penis. If the penis is uncircumcised, pull back the foreskin. Unroll the condom all the way down to the base of the penis. There might be some condom left rolled up. It's always a good idea to use extra lubricant with condoms. This will reduce the chances of a condom breaking and also increases sensitivity.

If you can't use your hands, and your partner can't either, you can try the mouth trick. Obviously the person attached to the penis can't do this, the partner has to. It can be tricky and you need to be careful with your teeth. Practicing a few times with a dildo, cucumber, or banana may be reassuring. Some condom packages are easier to open than others. Because the tiny rectangular packages might be harder to remove the condom from, you might want to start with the square packets instead. If you can get the condom in your mouth, suck it into place with the reservoir tip facing your throat. Have your lips or teeth closed enough so that the rolled edge doesn't go into your mouth—this is definitely not worth suffocating for. Use your tongue to press the tip toward the roof of your mouth behind your top teeth, so you are squeezing the tip against the back of your teeth and keeping air out of it. Using your lips and mouth, slide the condom onto the head of the penis or dildo. If you can, use your neck muscles to push the condom down onto the penis or dildo. If not, maybe your partner can move his penis toward your mouth. Once the condom is on a little, you can try to use a different part of your body to further roll the condom on. You don't need as much manual dexterity for this, so you might be able to use your hand, or your forearm or tongue.

Removing a Condom

Taking off the condom is as important as putting it on. If neither of you can use your hands, it may be best to pull out before or during ejaculation. If one person can get their hand around enough of the penis to hold the condom on, then you can wait until after ejaculation. A condom will fall off a flaccid penis, so it is important to withdraw the penis right after ejaculation before it becomes soft. Hold the condom at the base of the penis with your thumb and forefinger in a ring. Pull the penis out and move away from your partner. Either person can help with this. Slide the condom off and tie the end of it. If you can't tie it, have a plastic bag handy to throw it in right away. Don't flush it down the toilet. Don't let the condom or the penis touch your partner's genitals. Wash the penis before letting your genitals touch again.

If a condom comes off or breaks during vaginal or anal penetration, get the condom out right away. The partner shouldn't douche. Men might be able to protect themselves a bit by going to the bathroom and peeing and washing their genitals. A broken condom is a good reason to get STI testing. For women who are not otherwise protected against pregnancy, emergency contraception is available that can be taken up to seventy-two hours after intercourse, although the sooner it is taken, the better.

Dental Dams

Used by dentists during oral surgery, dental dams are thin squares of latex that can also be used to provide a barrier during oral/vaginal and oral/anal contact. Many sex educators recommend using dental dams, but no one knows how often they actually get used in real life. There is no good answer as to whether they should always be used for cunnilingus. The risk of transmission of HIV in this activity is lower than for fellatio or for penetrative sex, but other STIs can be transmitted fairly easily through cunnilingus. Because analingus also carries a risk of transmitting intestinal parasites, dams are a good idea. Dams can be tricky to use because they don't stay in place themselves and require a hand to hold them there. Some companies sell "dam garters" that you can wear to hold a dental dam in place. If you'd rather not pay for something like that, you can try cutting holes in your underwear and wearing them with a dam in place. People also sometimes use household plastic wrap instead of spending money on dental dams. It is not certain whether this is an effective barrier, but if you are using plastic wrap be sure to use regular wrap and not the microwaveable kind (which is more porous and less effective). With any sort of barrier, using some lube on the vulva under the dam will increase sensation. Dams and other barriers should not be reused. There are now nonlatex dental dams available for people with latex sensitivies.

Gloves

For any penetration play involving fingers and orifices you can use gloves. They are always recommended to cover a finger or fingers going into the anus, but they can also be used if someone knows they have HIV or an STI and their partner will be touching their genitals. Cuts or sores on the hands can increase the risk of transmitting HIV or hepatitis in either direction, and gloves can prevent this. Even if neither partner has an STI, gloves are a great way of keeping things clean and smooth (hangnails, small cuts on the fingers, and rough nails all get smoothed out when you put on a glove). The most common gloves available are latex gloves. People with latex allergies have several options. Two options are gloves made from vinyl and gloves made from a material called nitrile. Both provide protection and are still thin enough to transmit sensation.

Safety with Sex Toys

As with anything else, sex toys can be misused and have unpleasant or dangerous effects. In the allergy section in chapter 9, and later in this chapter, we talk about the materials that sex toys are made of. There are other safety considerations also.

Sex toys used for penetration may be harder than a real human being. They can have rough edges or seams that can cause cuts. Taking your time, using lots of lube, and paying attention to what you are feeling are all important.

If you have decreased sensation, then you need to be even more cautious. Use lots of lube. You may want to start off with a toy that is smaller than what you think you want, and then move up in size as desired.

> My girlfriend is a para and does not have a lot of sensation in her genitals. Once we tried a cheap dildo that didn't even look like a penis but had all these ripples so we thought it would do the trick. Because my girlfriend doesn't have sensation below the waist, she wasn't able to tell me that she was uncomfortable. We got a little excited and zealous with the dildo. Afterwards though, she told me that she didn't feel "right" for a few days. Her insides felt funny and she didn't want to use the dildo again for a while. I learned that I have to take it slow and that we might have to be more cautious if we are trying something that involves any kind of penetration.

For anal penetration, use only toys that are designed for this. A toy without a flared based can get sucked up into the rectum and will not always be easy to retrieve.

If you are going to use a cock ring, make sure that you will be able to get it off within thirty minutes, or that there is someone who can help you with this.

Autonomic dysreflexia (AD) is a potentially life-threatening response to a problem in the body that is most likely to occur in people with a spinal cord injury at or above thoracic level 6 (T-6). It is usually triggered by a bladder or bowel problem and by labor (the "having a baby" kind of labor). It may also be triggered by sexual activity, particularly the use of a vibrator. The body identifies a problem, but there is no conscious awareness of the problem because messages to and from the brain get blocked by the SCI. Blood vessels constrict and blood pressure rises. Other parts of your body sense the increase in blood pressure and try to counteract the change by slowing your heart rate and sending signals to tell your blood vessels to relax. These signals can't get through the spinal cord lesion. Blood pressure continues to rise.

The rapid rise in blood pressure can be very serious. There are ways to deal with AD, first among them learning the warning signs your body gives you and knowing how to check yourself out. Early warning signs are flushing, sweating, and increased spasticity. That's when you should get medical attention. More serious signs, which may occur later, are blurred vision, headache, nasal congestion, nausea, and erection of body hair. Having an emergency plan is crucial. Get into a position where your head is elevated, your clothes are loosened, and your shoes are off. Make someone stay with you while you or they call for help. For more information about AD the Paralyzed Veterans of America have put together an excellent, and free, information booklet. You can contact them at 888-860-7244, or online at www.pva.org.

Allergies

We come into contact with many materials during sex—soaps, deodorant, and perfume on our partner's skin; latex in condoms, gloves, and dams; rubber and additives in sex toys; spermicides and lubricants; and even traces of food on hands.

People who have allergies should keep in mind that they may react to something during sex. People who have never had an allergic reaction should consider this as a possible cause of pain during sex or of a rash that develops afterward.

In addition to allergies, people can have nonallergic reactions to chemicals they are exposed to. The most notable is that some people feel extreme skin irritation after exposure to some spermicidal foams or gels.

Latex Allergies

Most condoms, gloves, and dams are made of latex, as are many sex toys. Anyone who has had a lot of exposure to latex, especially to internal organs through multiple surgery or to mucous membranes through catheterization, is at a higher risk of latex allergy. People with spina bifida (menigomyelocele) often have latex allergies.

People with even mild latex allergies should avoid exposure to latex, as such allergies get worse with increased exposure to the substance.

Latex allergy can result in a rash, difficulty breathing, swelling, or even an anaphylactic reaction that can lead to death.

Condoms

At the time we are writing this book there are four brands of nonlatex condoms on the market. They provide protection from both unwanted pregnancy and STIs during penetration play. Condoms that are made from animal skin (called lambskin condoms) do protect against pregnancy, but do not provide STI protection.

Three of these condoms are the traditional male condoms. One is called Avanti and is manufactured by Durex. One is called Supra and is manufactured by Trojan. The last kind (see earlier sidebar) is called EZ-On. They are all made of a form of plastic called polyurethane. The benefit of this material is that it is very strong so the condoms are thinner than latex condoms. It also conducts temperature better than latex. However, polyurethane condoms are not as stretchy as latex condoms. For this reason the manufacturers have made these condoms a bit wider than the regular size of condoms. These condoms are still very expensive (about three times the price of latex condoms). We hope that as the market for this product increases the price will come down.

The Trojan Supra condom is only available with a spermicidal lubricant. Because some people react to the spermicide, you may want to try the Avanti instead. If the Supra is the only nonlatex condom available to you, you could try gently rinsing it off if you have had problems with spermicide before.

The other nonlatex condom is called Reality and it is a female condom. It is shaped like a male condom, only bigger, and is designed to be inserted in the vagina prior to penetration play. It has a ring that holds it in place inside the vagina and also comes out a bit to protect the surrounding vulva. This might give somewhat more protection against HPV and herpes than do male condoms. Because they haven't been around as long, we don't have any great tips about how to get one in without using your hands. However, it can go in a while before sex, so an attendant might be able to insert it before you and your partner get together. While the manufacturer does not support this, and we cannot recommend it, people are also using the Reality condom for anal sex.

Like the others, the Reality is much more expensive than latex condoms. It can also be noisy, with some people reporting a crinkly noise and others saying it can make farting sounds.

SEX TOY DISABILITY HISTORY

In an important piece of little-known disability cultural history, it was a man named Gosnell Duncan who in the early 1970s made the first silicone dildos for sale in stores. Gosnell was the president of his local chapter of the National Spinal Cord Injury Foundation and knew there was a need for high-quality toys for penetration play, as well as a market among people with disabilities. His company, Scorpio Products, was the first to make these amazing toys, and they are still widely available at high-end sex toy stores. Following Gosnell's pioneering efforts, a handful of companies now manufacture dozens of different styles and colors of high-quality, much safer dildos.

Sex Toys

There are different kinds of rubber, and most sex toys are not made of latex, as it is more expensive than other types of rubber. However, many toys are made in factories where latex is used for other things, and toys may be made in molds that were used to make latex toys. Someone with a severe latex allergy could react to these traces of latex.

Silicone is a safer material that contains no latex. Silicone has been used for medical purposes and has only recently been used for sex toys. Silicone toys can be boiled so that you can share them safely. Silicone toy manufacturers will inform you if latex was used in any part of the manufacturing process, something mainstream sex toy manufacturers won't do. Silicone is much more expensive than other materials used in sex toys, but it lasts longer so you won't have to replace your toy because it started to crumble.

All sorts of other ingredients, dyes, and scents are used in sex toys, and these can become problematic for people with allergies and environmental sensitivities. What's important is that you approach sexual products the same way you would food and other items you bring into your life. If the store you're purchasing from can't provide you with a detailed ingredient list, go to another store. Better stores and websites will already have ingredients listed for customers.

Sexual Coercion

It had been a long time since I had sex with a guy and I was really happy he wanted to be with me. It didn't seem to worry him that I couldn't move around as easily as other women. But when we got into bed he said I should go down on him. I didn't want to. He said no one else would want to have sex with me because I'm crippled so I should do what he wants. He kinda pushed me down but then he stopped, which was good because I would have bitten him if he had forced me.

Another part of sexual health and safety is being safe and free from coercion. A sexual partner who tries to get someone to do something they don't want to do sexually (like having penetration play without a condom) may use pretty slimy tactics to get their way. They may say things like "You are hopelessly old fashioned" or "I will leave you" or "You owe me so much that you should do whatever I want."

It is certainly fine for someone to ask for what they want, but that doesn't mean they are entitled to get it.

It isn't always women that this happens to. Men can also be coerced into sex acts, and often feel that they can't say no. They may think they won't seem masculine if they aren't eager to try any sex act or if they turn down sex.

In most relationships moments occur when one person really wants to do something that the other person isn't excited about. If the second person is willing, just not enthusiastic, it can be fine for them to go ahead and do it. But it isn't okay if that person really doesn't want to do it, but feels they should do it or are obligated to do it.

Sexual health and safer sex are attainable, and do not have to be messy or terribly inconvenient. What they are really about is a bit of planning and some imagination, as well as care for yourself and your health. You visualize what the issues might be and design a plan in advance that will give you what you need, and provide protection from what you don't.

13

Sexual Violence and Sexuality

Sexual abuse or assault is any unwanted sexual act, and could include touching, kissing, oral sex, and anal or vaginal intercourse. Some people also consider sexual harassment to be a form of sexual abuse. Sexual harassment can include someone making unwanted sexual comments, putting down someone sexually, or threatening to remove services if sex isn't provided. Commonly, unwanted sexual comments or touch may be made while someone is carrying out caregiving duties. In Canada, for example, a man with a disability took his attendant to court because the attendant was inappropriately touching him while giving him a bath. Although the case was dismissed, it became an important one for the issues it raised about the frequency of this kind of abuse. Sexual abuse and assault can also occur within partnered, dating, or sexual relationships.

> I have been raped twice. The second time affected me much more than the first because I was twenty-seven when it happened and it really undermined my sense of myself as a powerful woman, whereas the first time I was nineteen.... Also, the first time was over really quickly, whereas the second assault went on for hours. The second time really turned me off men and sex in general for a few years. I felt very powerless and vulnerable and very bitter about trusting anyone with my body. I was pissed off that I had been taken advantage of by someone much bigger and stronger than me and felt my body had let me down again. I didn't report either event to anyone but friends as I knew the whole police and court thing would be very humiliating, especially being disabled. I was terrified that police and the courts might think I should be grateful for the fuck and that they would be unable to believe me. I just gave up on sex for quite some time and my next affairs were very much controlled by me—no penetration, and I picked very gentle, trustworthy people to play with.

After being abused or assaulted we may be left with many feelings and responses about what happened that can linger and stay with us for years.

> I was molested as a child of ten, didn't remember until age twenty. I didn't learn to relax enough to orgasm until age twenty-eight, I think that was because of the abuse.

The effects of the abuse are not always related to the type of abuse, and vary from person to person. What may appear to one person to be a harmless touch could have profound meaning and consequences for another. At the same time we've come to think of sexual abuse as so bad that no one will ever recover from its effects, or that anyone who is doing all right after abuse or an assault is in denial. This is also not true. The responses to abuse can be as varied as the ways people find to move through it. This chapter is general in nature, and it is not our intention to discuss in detail the diverse range of experiences people have after sexual assault. For more information, please refer to the resources listed in the Sexual Assault Resources section of Chapter 14.

Why the High Risk?

I think disability is one means of singling out people for abusive treatment.

While researchers have recently begun to focus attention on collecting information on the risk of sexual assault in general, little information is available on the risks for people living with disabilities. The studies that have been conducted make it clear that there is a much higher than average risk of sexual abuse for people living with disabilities. The numbers from different studies vary, but the risk for women with disabilities is anywhere from two to ten times greater than that found in the general population. The risk is higher for men also, but the information we have on this is even more scarce than for women.

People living with disabilities are also at higher risk for other types of abuse. This may include physical abuse, financial exploitation, neglect (denial of food or personal care), denial of opportunities that may be taken for granted by others, and exploitation for medical or treatment purposes. This kind of exploitation occurs when a procedure is done that is not in the best interests of the person but instead for the convenience of an institution or caregiver.

Why are people with disabilities at higher risk of sexual assault? To start with, we are exposed numerous times to people we do not know and who are responsible for our care. This can occur at an early age for many children living with disabilities and may occur more often than for nondisabled kids. Most children are in the care of their parents, but children living with disabilities are more likely to be with other unrelated adults outside of their parents' presence. These may include hospital porters, volunteers, bus drivers, teaching aides, technicians, and others. As a result, potential abusers see that access to someone with a disability is easier than to other children. Perpetrators also may see disabled children as potential victims because they will remain silent or will not be believed in the event that they tell of the abuse.

Living with disabilities as children, many of us learn that we must be passive, compliant, and accepting of what is happening. We learn that it is easier to get the things we need or want when we do as we are told. This might be considered a form of institutional compliance—which occurs when people learn that by complying they can get their physical and emotional needs met. Institutional compliance is usually supported by the social service agencies we use or the places where we live, which often have written and unwritten rules to monitor our behavior and actions.

No one rewards a child for refusing a treatment or kicking up a fuss when they are being pushed around. By the time they are abused, many children know that you don't protest or fight when feeling humiliated, being pushed around, or made to feel uncomfortable. We may have also learned that turning to our parents in these situations often doesn't help, for we may not be believed. We may even come to think that the abuse was our fault. If we've grown up having been exposed to numerous procedures or treatments, it's very likely that our bodies have been touched and probed by many doctors, nurses, technicians, and other health care providers. As well, if we use caregivers to assist with the carrying out of personal care routines such as catheterizations and other intimate procedures, it may not be easy for us to distinguish between this institutional intrusiveness and abuse. By allowing children to be pushed around and to have their rights ignored for the greater good of "treatment," we increase the chances that they will be set up to be victims, as some of us were. We are not suggesting that this is intentional on the part of parents or service providers, but it's a built-in part of how our health care system works.

Some people in our society still see those of us living with disabilities as "damaged goods," not quite whole. An abuser may feel they can more easily convince someone that they deserve to be abused based on this.

The abuser might feel that no one would believe a complaint against them, because why would anyone want to assault someone who is already considered to be "damaged" in some way. The abuser may even justify to themselves that the disability makes it okay to abuse. It's hard to believe that someone would do that to somebody who is already considered vulnerable. This is another reason abusers get away with the abuse.

There exists a perception that people who live with cognitive and developmental disabilities lack the awareness of things that are happening. An abuser may feel that they can get away with the abuse because their victim won't know what's going on anyway. Again, this may also help to justify the abuse for the perpetrator.

Family members may see disclosure of sexual abuse or assault as a means of getting attention. People may be aware that some of us who have disclosed, reported, and laid charges have not been viewed as credible witnesses by the legal system.

Who Abuses?

We can't pick out abusers by how they look or what job they hold. We do know that the majority of perpetrators are men. Although there are a number of occupations that seem to have more abusers (the clergy, coaches, youth group leaders), most people are not abusers. Most who have been abused knew the abuser before it happened. They are family members, friends of the family, caregivers, babysitters, service providers. The risk for abuse increases as the number of people who are involved in our lives increases. People with more than one disability are often at higher risk, probably because of an increased number of service providers. People living with disabilities are also assaulted by people we don't know, but this is not as common an occurrence as abuse by people we do know.

Sexual abuse or assault can occur within a "romantic" relationship. When we give consent to have sex with someone once, or even one hundred times, we are not giving consent for any time they want to have sex.

I was dating this guy for a while. One night while I was sleeping, I woke up suddenly to find him trying to have sex with me—I wasn't even awake! His excuse was because I had "wanted it" before, he figured I would want it anytime...that I would always say, "yes." I didn't say "yes" this time. Although I ended the relationship, I kept trying to think if there was anything that I had done...I blamed myself for some time afterward. I felt really violated and distrustful of male partners after that.

Sexual assault within a relationship often coexists with other kinds of abuse as well as with alcohol or substance use. Those of us in abusive relationships may feel we have no options. It can seem impossible to leave a situation where we are financially dependent on our abuser. Social isolation is another factor in this. Women in abusive relationships have often been cut off from friends, family, and other supports. There may be physical barriers to getting away. Emergency services may be difficult to access. Even getting to the service may present problems if we have to make our travel arrangements several days in advance and can only visit the service during certain hours. Many emergency services are not able or willing to accommodate people with additional needs.

Men who are abused often feel they cannot tell anyone because there is still a belief that men want to have sex all the time and that they can't be forced into sex. Traditional gender roles (including the idea that men must be strong and take care of themselves) can also prevent men from speaking about abuse. Feelings of shame may be associated with the victim's not being able to prevent the abuse. If a man is abused by another man, he may fear that the abuse has made him gay.

The way we communicate may make it harder for some of us to give information about abuse or assault. We may never have the chance to disclose the abuse if the abuser is our primary support worker and goes with us to appointments. We may also not know the words or have the vocabulary to describe what's been done to us.

Reporting of abuse or assault is essential and crucial, but is not easy. Support services must be in place so that the person who reports abuse is not at further risk. If the abuser is a support person, they must be dealt with and replaced before the person returns home. If it is a relationship partner, the person may not be able to return home, particularly if the partner is the one who is the primary caregiver, cares for the children, or actually lives in the same residence as the victim. Group homes and institutions must have protocols protecting residents when they disclose abuse.

What Happens as a Result of Sexual Abuse or Assault?

I am a survivor of incest and medical abuse. The only effect that I think it had on the development of my sexuality is that while society was telling me that I was not a sexual being because I was disabled, I knew better because my father and others were treating me sexually.

It is hard to express myself sexually because of abuse.

I was sexually assaulted when I was twelve by a missionary. He and I were close and I told him I had a crush on another missionary. When it happened I was pinned down. I have allowed other men to abuse me but not to the same extent as that man. Most times I have a hard time getting it up with another man. Masturbation is easy, but it is hard to relax when a man wants to do me. I am slowly learning about what I like sexually. Communication is an issue. But recently I have had a good sexual experience. So now I know what a good sexual experience is. So I think I will have a hard time going back to my old ways of enduring bad sex with partners I am not attracted to. In the past I thought that I did not deserve a partner I found attractive. That I had to settle for what I could get, 'cause that is what someone like me has to do. I now know I was wrong.

People who have been sexually abused as children commonly experience feelings of alienation and isolation. They may feel different, or describe feeling outside the realm of being human. An experience of "differentness" is common for people with disabilities, even those of us who haven't been abused. Many of us have experienced devaluing attitudes toward our disability or health condition. As a result, we may have feelings of shame, abnormality, and nonbelonging. These may compound similar feelings that arise from being abused. We may come to believe that we are not like our "nondisabled" peers in terms of life experience. We may see ourselves as being different from them sexually and attribute it to the disability instead of to the assault.

> When I first started talking about the assault, it was in a group with other survivors. I was the only one with a disability. For the longest time I believed that the feelings of shame and guilt associated with the rape were because there was something about "me" that caused this to happen. I didn't know of other women with disabilities who had gone through similar experiences.... I felt so alone. I figured it was because of my disability and that I was somehow "deviant" and that's why I deserved it. After hearing from the other women in the group, I began to think differently and saw that it wasn't just because of my disability.

Trauma is physical or emotional damage that is the result of being hurt by something or someone. Trauma is experienced differently by all of us, and no one's experience of the event is exactly the same as anyone else's. Disability and how we have experienced our disability also have an impact on the experience of trauma and the process of healing.

> When I started looking at the abuse in my life, it wasn't always easy to figure out whether the feelings of hatred I felt about myself was because of the abuse or because of how I was treated by my family because of my disability. I couldn't separate them because it felt like they were linked to one another. Finally, I'm able to see that I have a right to feel safe. But at times, it is still a challenge to see that I am entitled to other rights, like the right to be treated with

dignity and respect, which is probably related to how I see myself as someone with a disability.

Some of you reading this have been sexually abused or assaulted. You may not have told anyone. Or you may be working with a counselor or therapist to help deal with the effects of the trauma. You may be ready to explore or consider how the violence can affect your sex life and sexuality.

There are some effects that many people commonly report as a result of being abused or assaulted. General effects include difficulty falling asleep, poor concentration, and feeling removed from your body. Flashbacks are vivid memories of the event or events. It is as if the experience is happening again. Flashbacks can be triggered by a smell, sound, or sight; by the time of day; or for no obvious reason. They are often accompanied by a fast heart rate and sweating, and can be triggered by sexual acts, including masturbation and fantasy. Other sexual effects include feeling mistrustful of potential sexual partners, a fear of being touched, guilt about sexual enjoyment, difficulty having orgasms, decreased sexual desire, and problems talking about sex.

Even without flashbacks you may have a feeling of dread or terror when you find yourself in a sexual situation. It can be difficult to stay present when making love with someone instead of retreating to a safe mental place.

> *I myself was not molested as a child. However, about nine years ago, I learned that my sister, with whom I'm very close, had been molested by our father as a child. That revelation escalated the fears I already had about sex. In fact, for months after learning about the incest, I couldn't bear to be touched by almost anyone at all, and had to stop my friends from trying to hug me.*

After sexual assault, you may experience a range of feelings related or connected to sexual pleasure, some of which may be conflicting. Some people might feel numb or only pain, while others may feel sexual arousal or experience orgasm. Feelings of fear, disgust, anger, shame, confusion, and betrayal can be intertwined with positive feelings. People may feel guilty about experiencing sexual pleasure. Some abusers try to make their victims feel sexual pleasure. This helps them justify what they are doing. They also think, that way people will be less likely to tell about the abuse. They may say, "See, you really did want it." It can be devastating to experience pleasure or an orgasm while being assaulted. We may feel that our body has betrayed us. We may feel that the assault is our fault, try to minimize its effects on us, or come to believe that it isn't really an assault. We may feel angry with our bodies for having a sexual response during a negative experience.

One of the worst things about an assault is loss of control. As a result of having suffered an assault, some people feel the need to be totally in control of every other aspect of their lives.

Years later, I see how affected I am by the abuse. I don't like surprises...I don't like being caught off guard. Once my friend tried to throw me a surprise birthday party and I froze. I disappeared somewhere "safe" and couldn't stay at my own party. Luckily there was someone there who I trusted and she helped me get a ride home with the accessible cab. I was totally overwhelmed by old feelings of fear and terror, like when I was a little kid and wasn't sure when my father would come in at night.

Feelings of self-hatred and worthlessness are common, and may become even further enmeshed when living with a disability or physical "difference." Some people feel they are "too damaged" to be able to ever have a sexual life.

There can be physical effects of an assault as well. Sexually transmitted infections, including gonorrhea, chlamydia, hepatitis, HIV and human papilloma virus, and herpes can all be transmitted during an assault. Pregnancy can occur. Vaginal or anal tissues can be damaged. It is important to be checked for these physical problems, even though physical examinations, particularly pelvic and rectal exams, may be difficult to go through. Having a supportive friend or counselor with you during an exam may be helpful.

What Can I Do to Have a Healthy Sexuality?

Healing takes place on many different levels. Regardless of whether you are celibate, dating, or in a relationship that is short-term or long-term, it is possible for you to heal sexually. It can take serious work to be able to reclaim your sexuality. Remember that the abuse was *not* in your control and was *not* your choice. It is possible to experience your sexuality in a different, positive way.

> When I am with a new lover I need to go really slow, moving from kissing to sensual touch to maybe penetration. It takes a long time for me to allow myself to trust new lovers—not only because of the abuse but also because of how I feel about my body, because my body doesn't quite fit the ideal of what a "normal" body should be. I've tried to really work on changing how I feel about myself and, for the most part, I've been able to stay focused. Sometimes I find that I fall into old routines when I feel vulnerable. I need to know that I can initiate sex and I can also stop it when I need to.

> I also endured a rape incident at the age of nine, while I was at summer camp. This, compounded with struggling with my sexual identity and my illness, has strengthened me. I have faced some hard times, but I am a survivor. My experiences and others give me hope about the resiliency of the human condition. I am better able to extend a hand to others in need; a lot of times, I have been in similar predicaments to theirs. I must admit that it is difficult to enjoy sex at times because illness and the rape have made it somewhat harder to see positively. I generally don't like dildo penetration because a lot of times it hurts my belly. I masturbate with my hands and perform oral sex with female partners. I work at being more and more positive about these issues every day. There are many others out there who face similar paths, and I know that I am not alone.

Many people find it helpful to have someone to talk with about how they are feeling. This does not mean that you have to go over the actual abuse again and again. Some people find they need to talk about the abuse, others don't. There is no "right" way to feel. Some of us have very few effects of abuse or assault and do not need or want any counseling. This is okay.

If you have sexual effects, it is often a good idea to begin your recovery with masturbation, rather than having sex with someone else. With masturbation you have total control of what is going on and can go at your own pace.

You may experience flashbacks even when masturbating. Try not to panic. Flashbacks can provide valuable information about your experience of abuse and can give you a chance to release some feelings that you've held on to. If you are feeling panicked, open your eyes and try to ground yourself. Focus on something in your room that will allow you to connect with the present. Breathe slowly with a long exhale. Remind yourself that you aren't being abused now, it is you touching yourself, and you are in control. You have a right to touch yourself in a loving way, you deserve pleasure, you deserve to be touched the way you want to be touched. You deserve to heal. Orgasms may bring on a number of different feelings. Enjoyment may be mingled with fear or guilt. You may want to masturbate without having an orgasm. This may help you look forward to touching yourself. If you have been having difficulty achieving orgasm, this can take the pressure off for a while.

Feeling ambivalent or negative about our bodies is common for many of us living with disabilities or chronic health conditions. If we are living with our disabilities from birth, we may have learned from our families, nondisabled children, and other adults (including medical professionals) that our bodies are physically deficient, incomplete, or defective. If we underwent a lot of medical interventions and hospitalizations, we learn quickly that our bodies "do not belong to us." Our bodies are seen as something that has to be fixed or changed. We are not good enough as we are. If we are augmentative or alternative communication users, we may not have had the vocabulary to talk about our experiences. For those of us who are survivors of abuse or assault, these feelings can be compounded by seeing our bodies as "damaged" or "broken" because of the sexual violation we faced. You can do various exercises to help you see your body in a more positive light. You can find one thing about your body that you like every day and write it down. Find pictures of yourself that you like and put them up where you can see them. Make an attempt to believe people when they tell you that you are looking great, or when they compliment you. Try to notice the parts of your body that are not causing you pain or distress. If an abuser said negative things about how you look, challenge those statements by saying the opposite statements out loud. More resources are offered in the Sexual Assault Resources section of chapter 14.

> *Acknowledging how my body is changing to tolerate less stress or use was most important in learning that my goals can change from minute to minute during sex. This didn't deemphasize orgasm, but it did give me more fluidity during sex. That acknowledgment made it more comfortable to me to stop sex at any time for any reason. After I got to that point—primarily through struggling with my pain and limited mobility—I was better equipped to deal with the trauma of sexual and emotional abuse that kept me from having healthy sex. If I could stop sex because my joints were uncomfortable, why not stop sex because my soul is uncomfortable? This was tremendously important to my sexual healing. And, as a result, only a few months ago I really started being able to have an orgasm with a partner.*

Learning to say "no" to sex when you don't want it is a key element on your road to reclaiming your sexuality. If you're not able to, it is likely that the experience of abuse and the feelings associated with it will be repeated. Being able to say "no" means that when you say "yes" you really mean it. It gives you control and a sense of safety. We know that for many of us living with disabilities, learning to say "no" is not easy. The habit of compliance learned from an early age may compromise our emotional and safety needs.

There is more to who you are than sex. However, we may have learned that our purpose, for the perpetrator, is to provide sexual gratification for someone else. It's difficult to feel that we are worthy and deserving of so much more when that is the message that we've been exposed to. The perpetrator may have told us that we should be grateful for the sexual attention because no one else would love us because of our disability. All these messages can become deeply ingrained and can have a significant impact on how we feel about ourselves, our worth, and our ability to move toward being in relationships with ourselves and others.

You can make choices now as an adult. You can choose when and with whom to have sex. You can strive toward feeling safe when feeling sexual. Taking a break from sex is also a choice. It can be helpful to realize that thoughts about sex or the abuse do not have to dominate your life. If feeling sexual is too painful, you can concentrate on other things in your life and then revisit sexuality to see if the break has helped you get through some of the pain.

Sexual Exploration

Start any sexual exploration slowly. You might want to start by looking at your body, describing it to yourself. Stroke yourself in areas where you weren't touched during the abuse. Over time, touch yourself in areas that seem scarier, always giving yourself permission to stop when you need to.

Make a date with yourself. If this isn't possible because of privacy, imagine a place where you could pay attention to yourself in a relaxed and attentive way. What does this place look like? What textures are you feeling? What is the light like? There is no rush. Breathe slowly and try to stay focused on the sensations you feel as you begin to touch (or imagine touching) your skin. At first it may be difficult to stay connected and not "split" from your body. Practice at your own pace.

What about partners? It is possible to have a healthy sexual relationship with someone else. If you've been celibate for a number of months or years and are now moving toward having a sexual relationship with a new lover, take the time to look at the reasons for why you want to be in a sexual relationship. Communicating with your lover or partner can be challenging and scary, but in many ways can bring new possibilities to your relationship. Just as you may need to pace yourself when disclosing information about your disability and what that might mean about being sexual with someone else, you may also consider the need to pace yourself and set boundaries about what you are willing to disclose about your abuse. However, if you think you might have a strong reaction to sex, it is a good idea to talk to your lover. Ultimately, you have the choice about how much you wish to share with a partner. If you can, share with your lover what they can expect from you sexually. If you want to go slow, say so. If you've made a commitment to not engage in sex when you do not want to, tell them. It takes courage to put yourself out there, as it does when talking about sexuality and disability. Take your time getting to know your lover and feel that you would be able to say "no" before saying "yes."

Practice what you'd like to say to a partner. You can do this with yourself, maybe in front of a mirror. You can also do it with a counselor or a friend. Try to think of what your lover's reaction will be. Practicing will give you an opportunity to be clear about what you want them to know. What you communicate should bring you closer instead of putting distance between you. You are worth it. You deserve loving support.

In general, talking to someone such as a counselor can be helpful. It may not always be possible to find someone who has knowledge about disability and sexual abuse and how those experiences can be intertwined. But talking about one of these issues may afford the opportunity to gain insights to see other parts of your experience. Your insights can then be shared with your lover so that they can also have a greater awareness of what is happening in your relationship outside of being sexual with you.

Sometimes people who have been abused feel decreased desire and also feel undesirable. These two can be linked. You can start by making statements to yourself about the parts of you that you may be able to see as desire-worthy and then expand it from there. Try exploring your body even if it doesn't feel sexual to you. You may come to discover some new desire that might be scary. You have experienced someone else's desires being forced upon you, so desire is associated with a lack of control. Without consent, you met the needs of someone else and their desire was used against you. You may never have let yourself experience natural sexual feeling. This might be compounded by the fact that people with disabilities are not considered to have sexual feelings and desires. Thinking about what is desirable outside of having sex may be one place to start—knowing that you don't have to perform for anyone else. Remember also that you are in control. You can let yourself want anything, and that doesn't mean you will go out and get it. Desire isn't bad if we are able to feel like it's in our control.

Learning about consensual sexuality (by reading this book, for a start), opening yourself to desire, exploring your sexual response, and learning that you can be in control will lead you to a healthier sexuality in which sometimes it will even feel safe to allow yourself to be out of control.

Always remember that there are people who can help. If you are in a situation where you are being sexually victimized, you can take action. Abuse hotlines are available, although if using the phone is not possible you will need to find out which ones have TTYs or are able to offer alternative ways of communicating such as email. If the agencies that are mandated to help you are not accessible, someone from a disability organization may be able to act as an advocate to get what you need. There are excellent resources available for survivors of sexual abuse. Some address issues related to sexuality, disability, and sexual abuse. There are some good websites where survivors with disabilities talk about their experiences and suggest some excellent resources.

14

Resources

Sexuality touches so many aspects of our lives that it was hard to choose which resources to include from the substantial body of literature, as well as offerings from websites and organizations. To keep this section to a manageable size, we chose to leave out resources that are primarily academic; the only exception to this is a book about medications and sexual functioning. We have also left out the major disability organizations, because they are easily found and often the first places people contact for information or support.

We have divided this chapter by topic. Within each topic heading we have broken resources into three types: print resources, online resources, and organizations. Because so many exciting and useful new resources are now available online, we have included many of these. Be aware, however, that websites come and go, and over time they may find different homes on the Internet, or disappear entirely.

In most cases, resources specifically intended for the gay, lesbian, bisexual, transsexual, and queer communities are included under each subject heading, and their focus is mentioned where it applies.

An online version of this resource list can be found at: www.comeasyouare.com/resources. We will make every effort to keep this list updated, and we welcome your help and suggestions with additions to the list. You can email us at: cory.s@sympatico.ca.

Centers for Independent Living

Online

EnableLink
www.enablelink.org
Contains an extensive directory of disability resources in Canada, including centers for independent living listed by region.

Independent Living Institute
www.independentliving.org/index.html
The institute, based in Sweden, works with projects that promote opportunities for self-determination in everyday life for persons with extensive disabilities, in particular personal assistance users. Its website contains many useful links and information on independent living across Europe.

Independent Living USA
www.ilusa.com/index.htm
Website contains links and directories for independent living centers across the United States, in addition to disability news and other disability related resources.

Organizations

Association of Programs for Rural Independent Living
5903 Powdermill Rd.
Kent, OH 44240
(330) 678-7648
www.april-rural.org/
Lgonz21800@aol.com

Canadian Association of Independent Living Resource Centres (CAILC)
1104-170 Laurier Avenue W.
Ottawa, ON, Canada K1P 5V5
(613) 563-2581, fax (613) 563-3861, TDD (613) 563-4215
http://cailc.ca
cailc@magma.ca
CAILC is a national umbrella organization that consists of local autonomous Independent Living Resource Centers (ILRCs). Each ILRC is community-based and controlled by and for persons with disabilities. CAILC is run by the individual ILRCs and provides support, training, networking with both government and nongovernment organizations, and information dissemination.

Disability Culture, Activism, and Stories

Print

BOOKS: While these books don't necessarily focus on sex, sex comes up in many of them. Some of them may be out of print. We have included them because you may be able to find them at libraries and used bookstores or via Internet used-book search sites.

Anesthesia: Poems, by Kenny Fries (Advocado Press, 1996).

Basic Skills, by Anne Finger (University of Missouri Press, 1991).

Black Bird Fly Away: Disabled in an Able-Bodied World, by Hugh Gregory Gallagher (Vandamere Press, 1998).

Bob Flanagan: Supermasochist, by Bob Flanagan and Sheree Rose, ed. by Andrea Juno and V. Vale (Juno Books, 2000).

Body Remember: A Memoir, by Kenny Fries (Dutton, 1997).

Bone Truth: A Novel, by Anne Finger (Coffee House Press, 1994).

Carnal Acts: Essays, by Nancy Mairs (Beacon Press, 1996).

Deaf in America: Voices from a Culture, by Carol Padden and Tom Humphries (Harvard University Press, 1990).

The Disability Rights Movement: From Charity to Confrontation, by Doris Zames Fleischer and Frieda Zames (Temple University Press, 2001).

Disability Studies Reader, ed. by Lennard Davis (Routledge, 1997).

Diving Bell and the Butterfly, by Jean-Dominique Bauby (Vintage Books, 1998).

Encounters with Strangers: Feminism And Disability, ed. by Jenny Morris (Women's Press, 1999).

Exile and Pride: Disability, Queerness and Liberation, by Eli Clare (South End Press, 1999).

Imprinting Our Image: An International Anthology by Women with Disabilities, ed. by Diane Driedger and Susan Gray (Gynergy Books, 1992).

Make Them Go Away: Clint Eastwood, Christopher Reeve and the Case Against Disability Rights, by Mary Johnson (Advocado Press, 2003).

The Me in the Mirror, by Connie Panzarino (Seal Press, 1994).

Moving Violations: War Zones, Wheelchairs and Declarations of Independence, by John Hockenberry (Hyperion, 1996).

A Nearly Normal Life, by Charles L. Mee (Little, Brown, 2000).

The New Disability History: American Perspectives, ed. by Paul K. Longmore and Lauri Umansky (New York University Press, 2001).

No Pity: People with Disabilities Forging a New Civil Rights Movement, by Joseph Shapiro (Times Books, 1994).

Nothing About Us Without Us: Disability Oppression and Empowerment, by James Charlton (University of California Press, 2000).

Pain Journal, by Bob Flanagan (Semiotext(e), 2000).

Past Due: A Story of Disability, Pregnancy, and Birth, by Anne Finger (Seal Press, 1990).

Plant of the Blind: A Memoir, by Stephen Kuusisto (Delta, 1998).

Points of Contact: Disability, Art, and Culture, ed. by Susan Crutchfield and Marcy Epstein (University of Michigan Press, 2000).

Pushing the Limits: Disabled Dykes Produce Culture, edited by Shelley Tremain (Women's Press, 1996).

Ragged Edge: The Disability Experience from the Pages of the First Fifteen Years of the Disability Rag, ed. by Barrett Shaw (Advocado Press, 1994).

Range of Motion: An Anthology of Disability Poetry, Prose and Art, ed. by Cheryl Marie Wade (Squeaky Wheels Press, 1993).

Slow Dance: A Story of Stroke, Love, and Disability, by Bonnie Sherr Klein (Random House, 1997).

Staring Back: The Disability Experience from the Inside Out, ed. by Kenny Fries (Plume, 1997).

Waist-High in the World: A Life Among the Nondisabled, by Nancy Mairs (Beacon Press, 1998).

"What Happened to You?": Writing by Disabled Women, ed. by Lois Keith (New Press, 1996).

Why I Burned My Book and Other Essays on Disability, by Paul K. Longmore (Temple University Press, 2003).

With Wings: An Anthology by and about Women with Disabilities, ed. by Marsha Saxton and Florence Howe (Feminist Press, 1993).

Women with Disabilities: Essays in Psychology, Culture, and Politics, ed. by Michelle Fine and Adrianne Asch (Temple University Press, 1990).

MAGAZINES: Many of these magazines run articles about sexuality, and you can access some information online free from their websites as well.

Abilities
340 College St., Suite 650
Toronto, ON, Canada M5T 3A9
(416) 923-1885, fax (416) 923-9829
www.enablelink.org

Kaleidoscope
United Disability Services
701 South Main St.
Akron, OH 44311
(330) 762-9755, TTY (330) 379-3349
www.udsakron.org

Mainstream Magazine
www.mainstream-mag.com

Mouth
61 Brighton St.
Rochester, NY 14607
www.mouthmag.com

New Mobility
No Limits Communications Inc.
P.O. Box 220
Horsham, PA 19044
www.newmobility.com

The Ragged Edge (formerly *The Disability Rag*)
For more information write to:
P.O. Box 145
Louisville, KY 40201
www.ragged-edge-mag.com

Online

Crip Commentary
www.cripcommentary.com
The "whenever" regular Web column of disability activist, writer, and poet
Laura Hershey. Full of insight, humor, and stuff to get really angry about, her
commentary is not to be missed.

Disability World
www.disabilityworld.org
A new webzine dedicated to advancing an exchange of information and
research about the international independent living movement of people with
disabilities.

Films Involving Disabilities
www.disabilityfilms.co.uk
A very thorough site that lists 2,500 feature films which depict or discuss disabilities. You can search on terms (like sex) to find films either by subject matter or by disability.

GnarlyBone News
GnarlyBone@aol.com
A semiregular free online newsletter published by Cheryl Marie Wade. To subscribe or unsubscribe email to GnarlyBone@aol.com with your request and
email address in the body of the email. Submissions are welcome; shorter is
better but not mandatory. Use black type on white background in no smaller
than twelve point.

Institute on Disability Culture
www.dimenet.com/disculture
Not updated regularly. The institute's mission since 1994 has been to promote
pride in the history, activities, and cultural identity of individuals with disabilities throughout the world. The purpose of this site is to provide information
about and share examples of disability culture.

London Disability Arts Forum
www.ldaf.net
A disability-led organization focused on promoting disability arts and the work
of artists living with disabilities.

On a Roll Radio
www.onarollradio.com
The first and only live weekly syndicated commercial radio talk show on life
and disability.

Organizations

Disability Advocates of Minorities Organization
DAMO's purpose is to represent, promote, and celebrate the abilities of disabled people of color through the encouragement and development of public education, public awareness, self-advocacy training, networking, artistic expression, awareness training, and consulting.
c\o Mission Council
820 Valencia St.
San Francisco, CA. 94110
www.sfdamo.freeserves.com
sfdamo@yahoo.com

Not Dead Yet
A national disability rights group opposing the legalization of physician-assisted suicide.
Progress CIL
7521 Madison St.
Forest Park, IL 60130
(708) 209-1500, fax (708) 209-1735, TTY (708) 209-1826
www.notdeadyet.org

Gender, Queer, and Transsexual/Transgender Resources

Print

Body Alchemy: Transsexual Portraits, by Loren Cameron (Cleis Press, 1996).

Exile and Pride: Disability, Queerness and Liberation, by Eli Clare (Consortium Books, 1999).

Gender Outlaw: On Men, Women, and the Rest of Us, by Kate Bornstein (Vintage Books, 1995).

The Last Time I Wore a Dress: A Memoir, by Daphne Scholinski (Riverhead Books, 1997).

Miss Vera's Finishing School for Boys Who Want to be Girls, by Veronica Vera (Doubleday, 1997).

My Gender Workbook: How to Become a Real Man, a Real Woman, the Real You, or Something Else Entirely, by Kate Bornstein (Routledge, 1997).

Pomosexuals: Challenging Assumptions About Gender and Sexuality, ed. by Carol Queen and Lawrence Schimel (Cleis Press, 1997).

Restricted Access: Lesbians on Disability, ed. by Victoria Brownworth and Susan Raffo (Seal Press, 1999).

Sex Changes: The Politics of Transgenderism, by Patrick Califia (Cleis Press, 1997, 2003).

Womyn's Braille Press
www.concentric.net/~tbraille/wbp/contents.htm
This publisher has been producing feminist literature on tape and in braille, with the help of dozens of volunteers, for nearly fifteen years. Its catalog contains more than 800 books. The titles are available in the United States through the National Library Service for the blind. If you are not registered with the NLS program, but have a print reading disability, contact WBP at (800) 424-8567 to enroll in the program and locate your nearest NLS library.

Online

Bent
www.bentvoices.org
A website for and about "cripgay men."

Deaf Queer Resource Center
www.deafqueer.org
A nonprofit resource and information center that provides information and resources to and about the deaf lesbian, gay, bisexual, and transgendered community. The website also has an associated IRC chat space and offers personal home pages.

Disabled Women on the Web
www.disabledwomen.net
Established by Corbett O'Toole of the Disabled Women's Alliance to provide information, resources, and support for women with disabilities to continue to change the world.

Eminism.org
www.eminism.org
The website of writer, speaker, and activist Emi Koyama, filled with articles about disability, queer and trans politics, sex work, and much more.

Gender Links
www.songweaver.com/gender
An extensive collection of links to websites of transsexual and transgender resources.

Passing Twice
http://passingtwice.com
An informal network of gay, lesbian, bisexual, and transgender stutterers and their friends. The group meets every year at the NSP convention, and also holds workshops at other stuttering conferences around the world. In between, members keep in touch through a quarterly newsletter, an email list, and an annual mailing list.

Queering Diabetes
www.queeringdiabetes.org
If you're lesbian, gay, bi, trans, intersex, queer, or simply questioning and you're diabetic, or if you're a significant other, friend, family member, or ally of someone with diabetes, then this site is for you. Writings, message boards, links, and more.

Youth Resources
www.youthresource.com/community/deaf/index.cfm
Resources, stories, and information by and about the deaf GLBTQ community, with good information for youth as well.

Organizations

The Disabled Women's Network of Canada (DAWN)
P.O. Box 22003, Downtown P.O.
Brandon, MB, Canada R7A 6Y9
(204) 726-1406
www.dawncanada.net
dawnca@canada.com

Gender Education and Advocacy
A national organization focusing on the needs, issues, and concerns of gender
variant people.
P.O. Box 33724
Decatur, GA 30033
www.gender.org

International Foundation for Gender Education (IFGE)
(IFGE) is a leading advocate and educational organization for promoting the
self-definition and free expression of individual gender identity. They are an
information provider and clearinghouse for referrals about all things which are
transgressive of established social gender norms. They maintain a bookstore
online and publish a magazine.
P.O. Box 540229
Waltham, MA 02454
(781) 899-2212, fax (781) 899-5703
www.ifge.org

The Intersex Society of North America
4500 9th Ave. NE, Suite 300
Seattle, WA 98105
(206) 633-6077, fax (206) 633-6049
www.isna.org
info@isna.org
A public awareness, education, and advocacy organization working to create a
world free of shame, secrecy, and unwanted surgery for intersex people (individuals born with anatomy or physiology that differs from cultural ideals of
male and female).

Meeting People

Please note: Listings in this resource section do not necessarily mean we recommend the resource. The authors have not tried most of the places listed below. In some cases we have got referrals from friends and survey participants, but in other cases we know nothing about the service. As with anything else online, we suggest you proceed with some caution, particularly when someone is trying to sell you something.

Online Dating Services

Dating sites online have become big business in the past few years. Many of the larger and better-known sites (including www.match.com, www.kiss.com, and www.nerve.com) offer a great opportunity to browse through hundreds of personal ads, get ideas to write and post your own, and make contact with others. Below we've included some lesser-known sites that are disability specific.

Bent
www.bentvoices.org
An online magazine for and about "cripgay men." It also has a personals section.

Date Able
www.dateable.org
One of the more established online dating services specifically for people with disabilities.

PeopleNet
http://members.aol.com/bobezwriter/pnet.htm
Contains articles about sexuality and some about sex and disability, along with links to both heterosexual and gay dating sites plus personal ad sites.

Reach Out Magazine
www.reachoutmag.com
A web-based magazine and online dating service. You have to pay to access all areas of the site, but some issues of the magazine you can view for free. The full site contains live chat on its own private IRC server, online ads (personal or for sale items), and message boards.

Newsgroups and Email Lists

Thanks to several large sites and Internet service providers that provide free and easy access to starting your own newsgroup, there are now several newsgroups (or lists) devoted to disability and specific sexual topics. Below are two of the larger sites that house these groups. You can go to these sites and search by the topic of a discussion group.

http://clubs.yahoo.com
http://clubs.excite.com
www.queernet.org
www-unix.umbc.edu/~korenman/wmst/forums.html

Camera Obscura
www.hicom.net/~oedipus/index.html
This excellent site compiles a wide variety of sites related to blindness resources on the Internet. It offers an extensive list of email lists related to blindness and dating.

Reproductive Health

Print

Mother to Be: A Guide to Pregnancy and Birth for Women with Disabilities, by Judi Rogers and Molleen Matsumura (Demos Vermande, 1992)

Reproductive Issues for People with Disabilities, by Florence P. Haseltine (Paul H. Brooke, 1993)

Women with Physical Disabilities: Achieving and Maintaining Health and Well-Being, by Danuta Krotoski, Margaret A. Nosek, and Margaret A. Turk (Paul H. Brooke, 1996)

Online

The Genetic Cleansing Project
www.geneticcleansing.org
An excellent resource, providing links to websites, books, and news articles about reproductive technologies, genetic screening, and, as the site puts it, "the medical establishment's quest to cull the human herd."

Having a Daughter With a Disability: Is It Different for Girls?
www.nichcy.org/pubs/outprint/nd14txt.htm
Special gender issue of the National Information Center for Children and
Youth with Disabilities *News Digest.*

Parents With Disabilities Online
www.disabledparents.net
Providing information, support, and resources to parents with disabilities since 1996.

Organizations

Center for Research on Women with Disabilities (CROWD)
CROWD is a research center that focuses on issues related to health, aging, civil
rights, abuse, and independent living.
3440 Richmond Avenue, Suite B
Houston, TX 77046
(800) 442-7683, (713) 961-3555
www.bcm.tmc.edu/crowd
crowd@bcm.tmc.edu

Disabled Womens Action Network of Ontario
Offers information resources related to reproductive health and reproductive
rights within Canada.
TTY (705) 494-9078
http://dawn.thot.net/index.html
dawn@thot.net

Through the Looking Glass (TLG)
A disability community-based nonprofit national organization that has pio-
neered research, training, and services for families in which a child, parent or
grandparent has a disability or medical issue. Their site includes extensive
resource listings.
2198 Sixth Street, Suite 100
Berkeley, CA 94710
(800) 644-2666, (510) 848-1112, TTY (800) 804-1616
www.lookingglass.org

Sexuality: Disability-Specific Resources

Print

Many disability resource books now contain at least a page or two about sexuality. While it's seldom news to you, if you're interested in a particular disability or chronic illness you may find looking at those books first well worth a try We have included only books with sexual content, and magazines that frequently cover sexual issues.

Aan hartstocht Geen Gebrek, by Karin Spaink (De Brink, 1991).
An interesting collection of erotic photos of people with physical disabilities, with text in Dutch. It may be hard to find, but is available for sale in Europe.

Being Sexual: An Illustrated Series on Sexuality and Relationships, by Dave Hingsburger and Susan Ludwig, illus. by James F. Whittingham. Available through Sex Information and Education Council of Canada, 850 Coxwell Ave., East York, ON, Canada M4C 5RI; (416) 466-5304.

Bob Flanagan: Supermasochist, ed. by A. Juno and V. Vale (Re/Search Publications, 1993).

Dis-n-tangle
A 'zine covering a range of queer disability topics, co-created by Fran Odette.
50 Cowan Ave.
Toronto, ON, Canada M6K 2N4
dispride_zine@hotmail.com

Dykes, Disability, and Stuff
A quarterly newsletter devoted to the health and disability concerns of lesbians. It is also unique in the range of accessible media available: standard print, large print, audio cassette, braille, DOS disk, and modem transfer.
P.O. Box 8773
Madison, WI 53708
http://tps.stdorg.wisc.edu/MGLRC/Groups/DykesDisabilitiesStuff.html
dykesdisabilityandstuff@juno.com

Easy for You to Say, by Miriam Kaufman (Key Porter Books, 1995).

Enabling Romance: A Guide to Love, Sex, and Relationships for the Disabled, ed. by K. Kroll and E. L. Klein (No Limits Communications. 2001).

Illustrated Guide to Better Sex for People with Chronic Pain, by Robert W. Rothrock and Gabriella D'Amore. Available through 201 Woolston Dr., P.O. Box 1355, Morrisville, PA 19067; (215) 736-1266.

Intimacy and Disability, by Barbara F. Waxman, Judi Levin, and June Isaacson Kailes. Available through National Rehabilitation Information Center, 8455 Colesville Rd., Suite 935, Silver Spring, MD 20910; (800) 346-2742.

Intimacy, Sexuality and an Ostomy, by Gwen B. Turnbull. Available through United Ostomy Association, (800) 826-0826.

Living and Loving: Information About Sexuality and Intimacy. Available through Arthritis Foundation, P.O. Box 19000, Atlanta, GA 30326; (800) 283-7800.

Novel Approach to Sexuality and Disability, by Georgie Maxfield. Available through Northern Nevada Amputee Support Group, 3985 Warren Way, Reno, NV 89509; (775) 828-0885.

Pushing the Limits: Disabled Dykes Produce Culture, ed. by Shelley Tremain (Women's Press, Toronto, 1996).

Real Crip Sex, by Robert Mauro. Available through 257 Center Lane, Levittown, NY 11756.

Sensuous Heart: Sex After a Heart Attack or Heart Surgery, by S. Cambre (1990). Available through Pritchett and Hull Associates, 3440 Oakcliff Rd. NE, Suite 110, Atlanta, GA 30340; (800) 241-4925.

Sex and Back Pain, by L. Hebert (1992). Available though IMPACC, 1 Washington St., P.O. Box 1247, Greenville, ME 04441; (800) 762-7720, (207) 695-3354.

Sex on Wheels
A newly published 'zine intended to create an open forum for discussion through thoughts/opinions/stories about sex and disability.
alessia_19@yahoo.com

Sexual Concerns When Illness or Disability Strikes, by Carol Sandowski (Charles C. Thomas). Available through 2600 South First St., Springfield, IL 62794; (217) 789-8980, (800) 258-8980.

Sexual Function in People with Disability and Chronic Illness, by Marca Sipski and Craig Alexander (Aspen Publishers, 1997).

Sexual Politics of Disability: Untold Desire, by T. Shakespeare, K. Gillespie-Sells, and D. Davies (Cassell, 1996).

Sexuality after Spinal Cord injury: Answers to Your Questions, by S. H. Ducharme and K. M. Gill (Paul Brookes, 1997).

Sexuality and Chronic Illness: A Comprehensive Approach, by Leslie R. Schover and Soren Buus Jensen (Guilford Publications, 72 Spring St., New York, NY 10012; (800) 365-7006).

Sexuality and Fertility After Cancer, by Leslie Schover (John Wiley and Sons, 1997).

Sexuality and Multiple Sclerosis, by M. Barrett. Available through the MS Society of Canada, (800) 268-7582. See online resource below for link to the downloadable version of this book.

Sexuality and Spinal Cord Injury, by Sylvia Eichner McDonald, Willa M. Lloyd, Donna Murphy, and Margaret Gretchen Russert. Spinal Cord Injury Center, Froedtert Memorial Lutheran, 9200 West Wisconsin Ave., Milwaukee, WI 53226; (414) 259-3657.

Sexuality and the Person with Traumatic Brain Injury: A Guide for Families, by E. Griffith and S. Lemberg (F. A. Davis, 1993).

Sexuality and the Rheumatic Diseases: An Annotated Bibliography 1970–1982 (Arlington, 1983). Available through Arthritis Information Clearinghouse, P.O. Box 9782, Arlington, VA 22209.

She Dances to Different Drums: Research into Disabled Women's Sexuality, by Kath Gillespie-Sells, Mildrette Hill, and Bree Robbins (King's Fund Publishing, London, 1998).

Women with Physical Disabilities: Achieving and Maintaining Health and Well-Being, ed. by D. Krotoski, M. Nosek, and M. Turk (Paul H. Brookes, 1996).

Film

Double the Trouble, Twice the Fun
Directed by Pratibha Parmer. Produced by Women Make Movies. Available from Women Make Movies, 462 Broadway, #500 D, New York, NY 10013.
UK, video, 24 min., 1992.
www.wmm.com
(212) 925-0606

Sexuality Reborn
Produced by Dr. Craig Alexander and Dr. Marcia Sipski for the Kessler Institute for Rehabilitation. Available from New Jersey Spinal Cord Injury System.
U.S., video, 48 min., 1993.
www.kmrrec.org/KM/nnjscis/sexuality_reborn.php3
(800) 435-8866

Sick: The Life and Death of Bob Flanagan
Directed and produced by Kirby Dick. Available from Lions Gate Films.
U.S., video, 90 min., 1997.
www.lionsgatefilms.com

Toward Intimacy: Women with Disabilities
Directed by Debbie McGee. Produced by Nicole Hubert. National Film Board
of Canada. Available from The National Film Board.
Canada, video and 16 mm., captioned, 61 min., 1992
www.nfb.ca
(800) 267-7710

Untold Desire
Produced by Eva Orner. Available from Filmmakers Library.
Australia, video, 53 min., 1994
www.filmakers.com/indivs/UntoldDesires.htm

Online

Bent
www.bentvoices.org
A website for and about "cripgay men," although it seems to be expanding (or
trying to) so as to include other voices in the queer disability community. It
also covers disability art and culture, both gay and straight. Offers a personals
section as well.

Come As You Are: Disability Resources
www.comeasyouare.com/index.cfm?andFA=Info.Disability_Resources
A great resource for information on making sex toys accessible, plus links to
other sex- and disability-related sites.

Cystic Fibrosis and Sexuality
www.cysticfibrosis.ca/page.asp?id=67
Two downloadable brochures, one for adults, one for youth, about sexuality
and CF.

Disability and Sexuality
www.gimpsex.org
An excellent resource with lists of articles, places to meet people online, and
other online and offline resources.

Disabled Hellas
www.disabled.gr
A collection of disability- and rehabilitation-related articles and books in the Greek language. Contains a link to sexuality resources. This resource is also available in print.

Diverse City Press
www.diverse-city.com
The publisher of excellent resources for people with developmental disabilities and their care providers, with a focus on sexuality. Through this site you can get all of Dave Hingsburger's books, which we recommend highly.

Empowerment Zone
www.empowermentzone.com
A site filled with articles related to empowerment. Check out its subsection on sexuality for articles ranging from sex therapy and Tantric sex to online etiquette.

Gimp Girl
www.gimpgirl.com
Offers four discussion forums, along with links to other sex and disability resources.

Good Vibrations Web Magazine
www.goodvibes.com
A monthly collection of articles online that can be found on the Good Vibrations website. Contains a column devoted to sex and disability.

How to Get Virtually Screwed: Finding Yourself Sexually in the Online Underworld
www.mainstream-mag.com/gimpsex.html
An excellent online article by Douglas Lathrop about sex and disability.

Nerve Magazine: Sex and Disability Issue
www.nerve.com/SpecialIssues/sexAndDisability
An online sex magazine that put together this special issue about disability.

Practical Suggestions from the Outsiders Club
www.practicalsuggestions.org.uk/contents.html
An information website run by the Outsiders, a British organization. Contains suggestions on meeting people, having sex, building relationships.

Sex and Arthritis
www.orthop.washington.edu/arthritis/living/sex/01
A good overview article that discusses issues ranging from body image to positioning to emotional aspects of sex and living with arthritis.

Sex and Disability Bibliography from SIECUS
www.siecus.org/pubs/biblio/bibs0009.html
Annotated bibliography of books on sexuality and disability, prepared by Sex Information and Education Council of the United States. Very thorough, but a little out of date.

Sexual Health.com
www.sexualhealth.com
The most comprehensive online source for disability and sexuality information. This is the best place to start any search for information, resources, and support regarding sexuality.

Sexuality and Disability Webliography
www.bccpd.bc.ca/wdi/sex&dis.html
British Columbia Coalition of People with Disabilities provides this excellent and very recent (2002) collection of online, print, and video resources related to sexuality and disability. Covers a wide range of disabilities and chronic illnesses, as well as GLBT issues.

Sexuality and MS
www.mssociety.ca/en/help/publications.htm
An excellent online book about sexuality and multiple sclerosis. You can order a hard copy of the book through the MS Society of Canada (visit the website for contact information) or download the entire book free of charge from this link.

When a Man Is Interested In You Because You Are an Amputee: A Woman's Perspective
www.usinter.net/wasa/contents8k.html
An article by Lynn Brancato offering a female amputee's perspective on devotees.

Women With Disabilities Australia: Sexuality Articles
www.wwda.org.au/sexualit.htm
An interesting collection of essays and articles about sexuality, reproductive health, and sexual assault by women with disabilities.

Youth Resource
www.youthresource.com
Offers sex information related to identity, orientation, abuse, health, and more. Also has a section on deaf youth.

Organizations

The Association to Aid the Sexual and Personal Relationships of People with a
Disability (S.P.O.D.)
286 Camden Rd.
London N7 0BJ UK
Tel: 0171-607-8851

Outsiders
BCM Box Outsiders
London WC1N 3XX UK
www.outsiders.org.uk
info@outsiders.org.uk

SexAbility
2398 Yonge St.
Toronto, ON, Canada M4P 2H4
(416) 486-8666, ext. 248

The Speak Up Project
This group has developed picture and word vocabularies for people who use
augmentative and alternative communication. These include vocabularies for
communicating during a medical examination, as well as words about sex, sexually transmitted infections, HIV testing, reproduction, birth control methods,
and sexual abuse.
www.aacsafeguarding.ca

Sexuality: General Resources

Print
Few of these titles contain disability-specific information, yet they are good places to start getting information that you can adapt to your own needs and situation.

Anal Pleasure and Health, by Jack Morin (Down There Press, 1998).

Becoming Orgasmic, by Julia Heiman and Joseph Lopiccolo (Fireside, 1988).

Bi Any Other Name: Bisexual People Speak Out, ed. by L. Hutchins and L. Ka'ahumanu (Alyson Publications, 1991).

Big, Big Love: A Sourcebook on Sex for People of Size and Those Who Love Them, by Hanne Blank (Greenery Press, 2000).

The Big O: Orgasms, How to Have Them, Give Them, and Keep Them Coming, by Lou Paget (Broadway Books, 2001).

The Clitoral Truth: The Secret World at Your Fingertips, by Rebecca Chalker (Seven Stories Press, 2000).

Deal with It! A Whole New Approach to Your Body, Brain, and Life as a Gurl, by Esther Drill, Heather McDonald, and Rebecca Odes (Pocket Books, 1999).

Erotic Massage: Touch of Love, by Kenneth Ray Stubbs (J. P. Tarcher, 1999).

Erotic Mind: Unlocking the Inner Sources of Sexual Passion and Fulfillment, by Jack Morin (Harper Perennial, 1996).

The Ethical Slut: A Guide to Infinite Sexual Possibilities, by Dossie Easton and Catherine A. Liszt (Greenery Press, 1998).

Exhibitionism for the Shy, by Carol Queen (Down There Press, 1995)

Fantasex: A Book of Erotic Games for the Adult Couple, by Rolf Milonas (Perigee, 1983).

Femalia, ed. by Joani Blank (Down There Press, 1994).

First Person Sexual, ed. by Joani Blank (Down There Press, 1996).

For Yourself: The Fulfilment of Female Sexuality, by Lonnie Barbach (Signet, 2000).

Full Exposure: Opening Up Your Sexual Creativity and Erotic Expression, by Susie Bright (Harper San Francisco, 1999).

Gay Sex: A Manual for Men Who Love Men, by Jack Hart (Alyson Publications, 1998).

The Good Vibrations Guide to Sex, by Cathy Winks and Anne Semans (Cleis Press, 2002).

The Good Vibrations Guide to the G-Spot, by Cathy Winks (Down There Press, 1998).

A Hand in the Bush: The Fine Art of Vaginal Fisting, by Deborah Addington (Greenery Press, 1998).

His Secret Life: Male Sexual Fantasies, by Bob Berkowitz (Pocket Books, 1998).

The Joy of Solo Sex, by Harold Litten (Factor Press, 1993).

Lesbian Sex, by JoAnn Loulan (Bookpeople, 1984).

Male Erotic Massage: A Guide to Sex and Spirit, by Kenneth Ray Stubbs (Secret Garden, 1999).

The Mother's Guide to Sex, by Anne Semans and Cathy Winks (Three Rivers Press, 2001).

Multi-Orgasmic Man: Sexual Secrets Every Man Should Know, by Mantak Chia and Douglas Abrams Arava (Harper San Francisco, 1997).

My Secret Garden: Women's Sexual Fantasies, by Nancy Friday (Pocket Books, 1998).

The New Male Sexuality: Revised Edition, by Bernie Zilbergeld (Bantam Doubleday Dell, 1999).

Pleasure and Danger: Exploring Female Sexuality, ed. by Carole Vance (Rivers Oram Press, 1993).

Public Sex: The Culture of Radical Sex, by Pat Califia (Cleis Press, 2000).

Sex for One: The Joy of Selfloving, by Betty Dodson (Crown Publishers, 1996).

Susie Sexpert's Lesbian Sex World, by Susie Bright (Cleis Press, 1999).

Trust: A Guide to the Sensual and Spiritual Art of Handballing, by Bert Herrman (Alamo Square Press, 1991).

The Ultimate Guide to Adult Videos: How to Watch Adult Videos and Make Your Sex Life Sizzle, by Violet Blue (Cleis Press, 2003).

The Ultimate Guide to Anal Sex for Men, by Bill Brent (Cleis Press, 2002).

The Ultimate Guide to Anal Sex for Women, by Tristan Taormino (Cleis Press, 1997).

The Ultimate Guide to Cunnilingus, by Violet Blue (Cleis Press, 2002).

The Ultimate Guide to Fellatio, by Violet Blue (Cleis Press, 2002).

The Whole Lesbian Sex Book, by Felice Newman (Cleis Press, 1999).

Women on Top: How Real Life Has Changed Women's Sexual Fantasies, by Nancy Friday (Pocket Books, 1993).

Online

Clean Sheets
www.cleansheets.com
A great place to go for online erotic writing, Clean Sheets was founded in 1998 by a small group of writers who dreamed of an online erotic magazine that didn't take itself too seriously, but still did its best to be fresh, clear, and exciting.

Scarlet Letters
www.scarletletters.com
One of the longest-running, women-owned, women-run, sex-positive webzines on the Internet, Scarlet Letters offers fiction and nonfiction writing, discussion forums, and plenty of art—all dealing with gender and sexuality from a "sex-positive" perspective.

Sexuality at About.com
http://sexuality.about.com
A site with essays and links to other sites offering a lot of "sex education" style information. This site contains an excellent essay by Linda Mona about sex and disability. It also has message boards and chat.

Society for Human Sexuality
www.sexuality.org
One of the best places to start any search for sex information online. It has articles reviewing sex toys, books, and dating services, as well as links to all sorts of sex-positive resources online. SHS sponsors events occasionally, mostly in the Seattle area.

Organizations

International Professional Surrogates Association (IPSA)
An organization that refers therapists and clients to surrogate partners who
have been trained by the organization. While they are not affiliated with any
professional college, the association maintains ethical guidelines and offers free
information and referrals to both clients and therapists.
IPSA
P.O. Box 4282
Torrance, CA 90510
http://members.aol.com/ipsa1/home.html
ipsa1@aol.com

The Sexual Freedom Coalition
BCM Box Lovely
London WC1N 3XX UK
www.sfc.org.uk/default.htm
mail@sfc.org.uk
A British organization devoted to reforming "Britain's silly old sex laws." Its
events often act as fundraisers for The Outsiders, and the organization is highly
inclusive of disability.

Sexuality: Health and Safer Sex

Print

The Black Women's Health Book: Speaking for Ourselves, ed. by Evelyn White (Seal Press, 1994).

The Clitoral Truth, by Rebecca Chalker (Seven Stories Press, 2000).

The Go Ask Alice Book of Answers: A Guide to Good Physical, Sexual, and Emotional Health, by Columbia University's Health Education Program (Owl Books, 1998).

The New Ourselves, Growing Older: Women Aging With Knowledge and Power, by Diana Laskin Siegal, Paula Brown Doress-Worters, and Wendy Sanford (Touchstone Books, 1994).

New View of a Woman's Body, by Federation of Feminist Women's Health Centers (Feminist Health Press, 1991).

Our Bodies, Ourselves for the New Century: A Book by and for Women, by The Boston Women's Health Book Collective (Touchstone Books, 1998).

Sexual Pharmacology: Drugs That Affect Sexual Function, by Theresa Crenshaw and James Goldberg (Norton, 1996).

Online

The Coalition for Positive Sexuality
www.positive.org
A grassroots, direct-action, volunteer group dedicated to providing teens with candid sex education materials. Some of the site is available in Spanish; contains limited disability resources.

Go Ask Alice
www.goaskalice.columbia.edu
Columbia University's health question-and-answer Internet service. A great place to ask questions and get answers on topics related to sexual health.

Immune Web
www.immuneweb.org
A website for people with fibromyalgia, chronic fatigue syndrome, multiple chemical sensitivities, and other conditions. A good place to go if you have questions about reacting to ingredients in sex toys.

Latex Information from the Spina Bifida Association of America
www.sbaa.org/html/sbaa_latex.html
Good information and links about latex allergies.

San Francisco Sex Information
www.sfsi.org
Toll-free (877) 472-7374; local tel: (415) 989-7374
A free information and referral switchboard providing anonymous, accurate, nonjudgmental information about sex. You can call it toll-free from anywhere in the United States.

Scarleteen
www.scarleteen.com
An excellent web resource providing straightforward sex-positive information for teens about sexuality and sexual health.

Organizations

American Association of Sex Educators, Counselors, and Therapists (AASECT)
A not-for-profit organization that certifies sexuality educators, counselors, and therapists. On request, AASECT will provide a list of certified sexuality therapists in a specific area. Send a self-addressed, stamped envelope to the address below.
P. O. Box 5488
Richmond, VA 23220
www.aasect.org

For a complete list of HIV/AIDS organizations in Canada contact:
Directory of Disability Organizations in Canada 2002/2003
Canadian Abilities Foundation
340 College St., #650
Toronto, ON, Canada M5T 3A9
(416) 923-1885, fax (416) 923-9829
www.enablelink.org
able@abilities.ca
Note: This directory is also available in many public libraries.

Ontario Sexuality and Developmental Disability Network c/o SIECCAN
A group of educators who work in the areas of sexuality and developmental
disability.
850 Coxwell Ave.
Toronto, ON, Canada M4C 5R1

Planned Parenthood Federation of America
This not-for-profit organization provides health care services, advocacy, and
educational programs on sexuality issues.
810 Seventh Ave.
New York, NY 10019
(800) 829-PPFA; to contact your local Planned Parenthood, call (800) 230-
PLAN or fax (212) 245-1845
www.plannedparenthood.org

Planned Parenthood Federation of Canada
A pro-choice, volunteer organization dedicated to promoting sexual and
reproductive health and rights in Canada as well as in developing countries
1 Nicholas St., #430
Ottawa, ON, Canada K1N 7B7
(613) 241-4474
www.ppfc.ca

Sex Information and Education Council of Canada (SIECCAN)
SIECCAN is dedicated to informing and educating both the public and professionals about all aspects of human sexuality, to support the positive integration
of sexuality into people's lives. May provide referrals to registered sex therapists.
850 Coxwell Ave.
Toronto, ON, Canada M4C 5R1
(416) 466-5304, fax (416) 778-0785
www.sieccan.org
Email:sieccan@web.net

Sexuality Information and Education Council of the United States (SIECUS)
SIECUS's mission is to affirm that sexuality is a natural and healthy part of living; to develop, collect, and disseminate information; to promote comprehensive education about sexuality; and to advocate the right of individuals to
make responsible sexual choices.
130 W. 42nd St., Suite 350
New York, NY 10036
(212) 819-9770, fax (212) 819-9776
www.siecus.org
siecus@siecus.org

Sexuality: Products (Toys, Books, Videos/DVDs)

Print

Good Vibrations: The New Complete Guide to Vibrators, by Joani Blank and Ann Whiden (Down There Press, 2000).

Good Vibrations Guide to Adult Videos, by Cathy Winks (Down There Press, 1998).

The Good Vibrations Guide to Sex, by Cathy Winks and Anne Semans (Cleis Press, 2002).

Sex Toys 101: A Playfully Uninhibited Guide, by Rachel Venning and Claire Cavanah (Fireside, 2003).

Online

WHERE TO BUY SEX TOYS
Hundreds of stores and websites offer sex toys for sale. Here we recommend only companies we have either purchased from or worked with directly.

Blowfish
www.blowfish.com
No retail store, but the website offers a unique and interesting online catalog. Good prices and very helpful service. No disability-specific information.

Bluedoor
www.bluedoor.com
(888) 922-4387
A website that will rent videos to people in any state of the United States. It carries a good selection of sex education titles and pornography.

Come As You Are
www.comeasyouare.com
701 Queen St. West
Toronto, ON, Canada M6J 1E6
(877) 858-3160, (416) 504-7934
5427 St. Laurent Blvd.
Montreal, QC Canada H2T 1S5
(514)-495-0444, fax (514) 495-0464
vtq@veneztelsquels.com
mail@comeasyouare.com
Great selection (sex toys, books, videos/DVDs), excellent service. This site also offers disability-specific information on adapting toys, plus links to other useful sites. Both retail stores are fully accessible, and one of the authors of this book is a worker-owner of this company.

Good Vibrations
www.goodvibes.com
1210 Valencia St.
San Francisco, CA 94110
1620 Polk St.
San Francisco, CA 94109
2504 San Pablo Ave.
Berkeley, CA 94702
(800) 289-8423
An excellent company, with three physical locations, a website, and a paper catalog. The Berkeley store is more accessible (with accessible washroom). Website contains helpful information related to disability. Also offers an online magazine that features a regular column about sex and disability. Also rents videos.

Liberator Shapes
www.liberatorshapes.com
Angular pillows designed for helping with sexual positioning.

Probe
One of the few lubricants that uses a natural preservative, Probe is manufactured by Davryan Laboratories. Their site offers detailed information about the product, places to purchase it, and contact information.
(800) 637-7623
www.davryan.com

The Stockroom
www.thestockroom.com
One of the oldest online places to buy sex toys, The Stockroom had an excellent reputation early on among blind computer users for their detailed text descriptions of all their products. They have a much larger selection of BDSM products than the other sites listed in this section.
(800) 755-8697

Toys in Babeland
www.babeland.com

94 Rivington St.
New York, NY 10002

43 Mercer St.
New York, NY 10013

707 E. Pike St.
Seattle, WA 98122

(800) 658-9119
Good selection and prices, friendly and helpful service. No disability-specific information.

Xandria Collection
www.xandria.com
165 Valley Dr.
Brisbane, CA 94005
(800) 242-2823
Many years ago Xandria produced a sex toy catalog specifically for people with disabilities. It has a few good tips, and it is great that the site made the effort to get the word out. Its prices are higher than many of the other sites and stores listed.

Sexuality: S/M and Fetish Resources

Print

Art of Japanese Rope Bondage, by Midori (Greenery Press, 2001).

Bob Flanagan: Supermasochist, by Bob Flanagan and Sheree Rose, ed. by Andrea Juno and V. Vale (Juno Books, 2000).

Deviant Desire: Incredibly Strange Sex, by Katharine Gates (Juno Books, 2000).

The New Bottoming Book, by Janet Hardy and Dossie Easton (Greenery Press, 2001).

The New Topping Book, by Dossie Easton and Janet Hardy (Greenery Press, 2003).

On the Safe Edge, by Trevor Jacques (Alternate Sources, 1993).

Screw the Roses, Send Me The Thorns, by Philip Miller, Molly Devon, and William A. Granzig (Mystic Rose Books, 1995).

Sensuous Magic: A Guide to S/M for Adventurous Couples, by Patrick Califia (Cleis Press, 2002).

S/M 101: A Realistic Introduction, by Jay Wiseman (Greenery Press, 1998).

Online

BDSM and Disability Discussion Groups
http://groups.yahoo.com/group/BDSM_4_PWD
http://groups.yahoo.com/group/disAbledpervs
Two Yahoo discussion groups that focus on discussions around BDSM and disabilities.

BRC BDSM Resource Center
www.thebrc.net
A collection of articles and links related to BDSM. There are several articles focusing on disability in the archives section of the site.

Fetish Diva Midori
www.fetishdiva.com
The main site for Midori, sex educator extraordinaire and Japanese rope bondage expert. This site links to her other two sites, one of which lists the workshops she offers across North America.

Kink Aware Professionals
www.bannon.com/kap
This site lists professionals (including therapists, doctors, lawyers, and others) who are aware of and sensitive to the needs of people who choose alternative sexual expressions like S/M.

Sexuality.org Resources on BDSM
www.sexuality.org/bdsm
An excellent place to start learning about BDSM, this site features articles on everything from negotiating a scene to finding partners, to specific play techniques.

Organizations

National Leather Association
www.nla-i.com
NLA International is one of the oldest and largest leather/BDSM/fetish organizations in the world. They have a sketchy history with disability, but the site is a good place to find out about events, local chapters, and information.

Sexual Assault Resources

Thanks to Wendi Abramson, Director of Disability Services at Safe Place for suggestions with these resources.

Print

Disability, Sexuality, and Abuse: An Annotated Bibliography, by D. Sobsey, S. Gray, D. Wellis, D. Pyper, and B. Reimer-Heck (Paul H. Brookes, 1991).

I Contact: Sexuality and People with Developmental Disabilities, by D. Hingsburger (Ida Publishing, 1990).

I Openers: Parents Ask Questions About Sexuality and Their Children with Developmental Disabilities, by D. Hingsburger (Family Support Institute Press, 1993).

No More Victims: A Manual to Guide Counsellors and Social Workers in Addressing the Sexual Abuse of People with a Mental Handicap, by M. Ticoll (Roeher Institute, 1992).

No More Victims: A Manual to Guide Families and Friends in Preventing the Sexual Abuse of People with a Mental Handicap, by M. Ticoll (Roeher Institute, 1992).

Serving Women with Disabilities: A Guide for Domestic Abuse Programs, by Leslie A. Myers (Center for Research on Women with Disabilities, Baylor College of Medicine, 1999).

Sexual Assault Survivor's Handbook: For People with Developmental Disabilities and Their Advocates, (R and E Publishers, Saratoga, Calif.,Baladerian, N.J., 1991).

The Survivor's Guide to Sex: How to Have an Empowered Sex Life After Child Sexual Abuse, by Staci Haines (Cleis Press, 1999).

Violence and Abuse in the Lives of People with Disabilities: The End of Silent Acceptance?, by Dick Sobsey (Paul H. Brookes, 1994).

Violence Against Disabled Women, by Barbara Waxman-Fiduccia and Leslie R. Wolfe (Center for Women's Policy Studies, 1999). This article can be downloaded for free at
www.centerwomenpolicy.org/report_download.cfm?ReportID=4
or by contacting the Center for Women's Policy Studies
1211 Connecticut Avenue, N.W. Suite 312
Washington, DC 20036
(202) 872-1770, (202) 296-8962

Violence Prevention Resource Guide for Women with Disabilities (Canadian Abilities Foundation, 2001).
340 College St., #650
Toronto, ON, Canada M5T 3A9
(416) 923-1885, fax (416) 923-9829
www.enablelink.org
able@abilities.ca

Working With Abuse Survivors: A Guide for Independent Living Centers, by Leslie A. Myers (Center for Research on Women with Disabilities, Baylor College of Medicine, 1999).

Online

Advocate Web
www.advocateweb.org
A nonprofit organization providing information and resources regarding abuse by "helping professionals." Their website has a section focusing on disability issues.

Canadian Women's Internet Directory
http://directory.womenspace.ca/Violence_Against_Women/Lists_of_Shelters_an d_Services
Contains a partial list of rape crisis centers across Canada.

Incest and Abuse Information from About.com
http://incestabuse.about.com
A good collection of links to websites and discussion groups about incest and sexual abuse.

Organizations

Education Wife Assault
A Canadian organization that informs and educates individuals and communities about the abuse of women. They offer disability-specific resources and training.
427 Bloor Street West, Box 7
Toronto, ON Canada M5S 1X7
(416) 968-3422, (416) 968-2026, TTY (416) 968-7335
www.womanabuseprevention.com
info@womanabuseprevention.com

Rape Abuse Incest National Network (RAINN)
635-B Pennsylvania Ave., SE
Washington, DC 20003
Organization that runs the National Sexual Assault Hotline, which can be contacted in the United States at (800) 656-4673.

Safe Place
An organization focusing on sexual assault and domestic violence, Safe Place has begun to offer their disability initiatives in the United States.
P. O. Box 19454
Austin, Texas 78760
(512) 356-1599, (512) 385-0662, TTY (512) 482-0691
www.austin-safeplace.org

Sex Work

Print

Real Live Nude Girl, by Carol Queen (Cleis Press, 2002).

Sex Work, ed. by Frédérique Delacoste and Priscilla Alexander (Cleis Press, 1998).

Tricks and Treats: Sex Workers Write About Their Clients, ed. by Matt Bernstein Sycamore (Haworth, 2000).

Turning Pro: A Guide to Sex Work for the Ambitious and the Intrigued, by Magdalene Meretrix (Greenery Press, 2001).

Whores and other Feminists, ed. by Jill Nagle (Routledge, 1997).

Online

Commercial Sex Information Service
www.walnet.org/csis/groups
A fine collection of news and links related to sex work, from Canada.

International Sex Workers Rights Organizations
www.swimw.org/orgs.html
Contains a list of organizations around the world working toward improving the rights of sex workers.

Why Disabled People Make the Best Clients
www.sfc.org.uk/adults/issue02/15disabl.htm
An article about sex work and clients with disabilities. Not an argument everyone will agree with, but an interesting article to read.

Yoga, Tantra, and Spiritual Sex

Print

The Essential Tantra: A Modern Guide to Sacred Sexuality, by Kenneth Ray Stubbs (Tarcher/Putnam, 2000).

Healing Love Through the Tao: Cultivating Female Sexual Energy, by Mantak Chia and Maneewan Chia (Healing Tao, 1991).

The Heart of Yoga: Developing a Personal Practice, by T. K. V. Desikachar (Inner Traditions, 1999).

Health, Healing and Beyond: Yoga and the Living Tradition of Krishnamacharya, by T. K. V. Desikachar (Aperture, 2001).

Multi-Orgasmic Man: Sexual Secrets Every Man Should Know, by Mantak Chia and Douglas Abrams Arava (Harper San Francisco, 1997).

Soul Sex: Tantra for Two, by Pala Copeland and Al Link (New Page Books, 2003).

Spiritual Sex: Ecstasy Through Tantra, by J. Mumford (Llewellyn Publications, 1987).

Tantra Spirituality and Sex, by B. S. Rajneesh (Rajneesh Foundation, Rajneeshpuram, 1983).

Tantra: The Yoga of Sex, by O. V. Garrison (Julian Press, 1964).

Taoist Secrets of Love: Cultivating Male Sexual Energy, by Mantak Chia and Michael Winn (Aurora Press, 1984).

Online

Tantric Sex: The Gift of Sexual Energy
www.paratetra.net/ustexts/sex/tantra.htm
This links to an excellent article by Mitch Tepper about spiritual sex and disability. Not to be missed.

Secret Garden
http://secretgardenpublishing.com
The website for Secret Garden Publishing, the company founded by Kenneth Ray Stubbs, an excellent teacher and author on spiritual sex.

Tantra.com
www.tantra.com
A good place to start online explorations about tantric sex. They push a lot of products on the site, but there is a lot of free information as well.

Universal Tao Center
www.universal-tao.com
The center run by Mantak Chia, considered to be one of the great masters of Taoist sexuality (and an author of several books included above). This site contains links to books, classes offered around the world, and other websites focusing on Taoist sexuality.

Glossary of Gender and Sex Terms

Because there is so much terminology involved in talking about sex and disability, we wanted to give you this quick resource to refer to basic definitions we use in the book. All definitions by nature are rigid, but we aren't. We are never just one thing, and just because a definition for how we feel or who we are doesn't exist, it doesn't mean there's something wrong with us. All discussions of sexuality and disability need to be seen in this fluid context. Terminology can change rapidly, and new words for who we are keep cropping up.

Gender

The term *gender* usually refers to the learned or socially constructed aspects of who you are as masculine or feminine. Sex is what we are born with, and gender is what we do with it. And for many people it is straightforward. But for a lot of us, gender is more complicated than that. Many of us don't experience our genders the way we're "supposed" to. For some of us, gender is fluid, changing over the course of a lifetime. We all are capable of change, and for many of us, desires change as we grow and discover more of who we are and what we are capable of feeling and doing. We can break our definition of gender into three parts: genetic gender, physical gender, and gender identity.

Genetic gender

Most people have, in every cell, two chromosomes that determine their *genetic gender.* A person with two X chromosomes is genetically female, and a person with an X and a Y chromosome is genetically male. But it is possible to have some cells with two X's and some with an X and a Y. Some people have only one gender chromosome (X). Some people have an extra chromosome (XXY or XYY). So even on a chromosomal level, there are far more than two options.

Physical gender

Our anatomy—our internal organs and the appearance of our bodies—most often matches our genetic gender, but not always. Sometimes baby girls are born with a very large clitoris that looks like a penis. This can be due to *congenital adrenal hyperplasia,* which is caused in utero by an anomaly of the adrenal glands. Or a boy might have a small penis with the urethra at it's base instead of at the end. This is called *hypospadias.* Genetic males whose bodies can't respond to testosterone will often have genitals that look like girls', even though they have testicles that produce male hormones.

Gender identity

What gender you *feel* you are also may or may not match your genetic or physical gender. So you may have been born with a penis and testicles but speak softly and love to wear dresses with yards of lace. Even though these attributes are usually associated with women, you still *feel* like a man. What if you feel more like a woman, but can't explain exactly why. Or what if you *are* a woman—and not a thing about femininity resonates with you personally. We would like to propose that the problem is with the limited options we are given—not with how we feel or the words we use to describe ourselves. There is intense social pressure to choose one *gender identity,* follow the rules, and never waver.

Sex

Sexual Behavior

This is what people usually mean when they say *sex.* Kissing, hugging, petting, gazing into someone's eyes (or your own), talking dirty, fucking, tickling someone with your foot, fantasizing—you name it, if you're doing it to arouse yourself or someone else, it's *sexual behavior.*

Sexual Orientation

Who do you want to have sex with? If you are mainly sexually attracted to people of the same gender, your *sexual orientation* is usually considered homosexual (gay, lesbian). If you are predominantly attracted to people of the "opposite" gender, your orientation is considered heterosexual (straight), and if you are attracted to both sexes your orientation is considered bisexual (bi, AC/DC).

Sexual Identity

Sexual identity is the most complicated of these three terms. It refers not to what we do, or who we do it with, but how we define our sexuality.

Our sexual identity is the way we see ourselves and define ourselves in relation to the rest of the world. It also encompasses the sexual behaviors we like, who we like to do them with, and more. Sexual identity also includes who we look to for intimate emotional support and who we choose as long-term partners, not just who we like to get hot with. For example, some men who are in long-term relationships with women have anonymous sex with other men. Most of these men would never call themselves gay or bisexual. Yet some people might say, "Oh, he's just in the closet, he isn't being true to himself." While this may be true for some men who have sex with men, it isn't for all of them. They may get their primary emotional, spiritual, romantic pleasure from being in relationships with women and ALSO like having sex with men.

Asexual

This term usually means "devoid of all sexuality." It's often applied to people who are not currently interested in sex or sexual behavior. We think *asexual* is a terrible term because we feel everyone has the potential to have sexual feelings. Even when we aren't being sexual or feeling sexual (either by choice or circumstance) we are still sexual beings.

Intersexed

Intersexuality is used to describe people who are born with sex chromosomes, external genitalia, or internal reproductive organs that don't match each other in the usual way. This is also sometimes called being born with "ambiguous genitalia." Not unlike the harmful "normalization" surgeries done on many people with physical disabilities for cosmetic reasons, doctors may advocate for newborn babies who are *intersexed* to receive plastic surgery to "correct" genitalia that simply don't look right (this could be mean a large clitoris, or a small penis). As adults, people who identify as intersexed have to contend with feelings about the surgery as they piece together a gender and sexual identity that feels right for them. Often they will have been raised being told they were a gender different than how they felt, and in many cases they will not be told the details about their surgery.

Pansexual

Everyone has their own definitions, particularly with new words like *pansexual*. Here's how we like to think of it. While heterosexual suggests your interest is towards the opposite gender, homosexual suggests the same gender, and bisexual suggests either gender, being pansexual means that you identify as having a sexual orientation towards all people potentially. It is a much broader term that would encompass being attracted to people who don't identify as either male or female. It may also suggest that you acknowledge that you could be sexually aroused by a beautiful painting, or the sound a babbling brook.

Queer

The word *queer* has come to be synonymous with "alternative sexual identity." Queer was originally a derogatory word used against people who were seen as odd (or worse) because of their sexual orientation. But it has since been reclaimed by gays, lesbians, bisexuals, and transsexuals (in the same way some disability groups have reclaimed "crip" and "gimp"). Now many people consider queer to describe a broader approach to sexual identity in which a person accepts a wide diversity of sexual practices (for example, S/M sex, polyamory, and fetishes) or has a sexual interest in a diversity of genders. Some use the term to describe a left-wing stance toward sexual politics. Others use the term because they just don't feel their sexuality fits into the heterosexual cultural norms that value marriage and monogamy over all else.

Transgendered

This is an umbrella term which encompasses people who feel that their lived gender differs from the "norm." *Transgendered* people may be transsexual (see below), or they may also cross gender lines in other ways. Transvestites (those whose gender identity includes *cross-dressing*, dressing in the apparel of the opposite sex), drag queens (who cross-dress to amuse, to entertain, or to make a political statement), butch (masculine identifying) and femme (feminine identifying) lesbians, and others identify as transgendered.

Transsexual

Transsexuals are people who identify as one gender but whose physical gender is that of the opposite gender. Male-to-female transsexuals (MTF for short) are born with the physical gender of men but identify as a female; and female-to-male transsexuals (FTM) are born with the physical gender of women but identify as male. People who are transsexual don't simply wish they were a different gender, they know they *are* that gender. They experience life as a gender different from the one they were born into. Transsexual people may be either heterosexual or homosexual.

Some transsexuals will undergo hormone treatment and/or sex reassignment surgery to alter their bodies to be more in line with how they feel inside. This process is called *transitioning*.

Index

A

ableism, 25, 31
accessibility, xi, 9, 21-22, 32, 64, 67, 74, 92, 94, 96-98, 102, 114, 117, 119, 130-131, 156, 189, 201, 210, 217-218, 221, 236-237, 250, 257, 264, 279, 283, 289
adrenal glands, 144, 330
African American, 210
AIDS, 260-261; *see also* human immunodeficiency virus (HIV)
alcohol, 55, 67, 142, 154, 279,
allergies, 105, 170, 198, 206, 252; latex, 143, 218-219, 255, 267-268, 269-270, 272
amyotrophic lateral sclerosis (ALS), 141
anal beads, 199-200
Anal Pleasure and Health, 174
anal sex, 102, 162-165, 169, 174-176, 177, 184, 274, 283; and lubricants, 205; and rectal surgery, 143; and safer sex, 220, 266-267, 271; and sex toys, 195-197, 198-200, 268; and STIs, 259-261
analingus, 164-165; and safer sex, 267; and STIs, 261
anemia, 130
Anne Johnston Health Station, xii
antibiotics, 258, 259, 262
antidepressants, 66-67, 137
anus, 40, 43, 45, 46-47, 119, 143, 157, 162, 165, 174-176, 198, 202, 220, 258, 267
anxiety, 52, 125-126, 134-135, 229
arthritis, 110, 117, 129, 144
asexual, 332
asthma, 125, 126
atenolol, 66
audio tape, 64

augmentative and alternative communication (AAC), 64, 71, 74, 82, 108, 285
autonomic dysreflexia, 149, 221, 269
Avanti, 270-271

B

back pain, 80, 159
baclofen, 66
bacteria, 176, 220, 258, 259, 261-262
bacterial infections, 204
Bartholin's glands, 41
bathhouses, 128
bathing, 105, 116, 142, 144, 153, 164, 218
BDSM, 237, 239; *see also* S/M
Bend Over Boyfriend, 169
birth control, 85, 146, 264, 266, 270
bisexual, xi, 19, 22, 86, 132, 212, 237, 291, 331, 333
bladder, 41, 43, 44, 56, 65, 81, 85, 142, 143, 144, 146, 147, 148, 151, 154, 209, 258, 269
Blake, Andrew, 213
blind, 76, 82, 237; *see also* visual impairment
blindfolds, 207, 244, 253
Bliss board, 82, 125
blood pressure, 33, 57, 269; *see also* autonomic dysreflexia
body image, 23, 113, 152-153
body mapping, 140
bondage, 207, 235, 239, 245, 246, 254
books, erotic, 209-211, 221-222; self-help, 15, 48; sex manuals, 31, 171, 174-175, 177, 235
bookstores, 210; adult, 221
boundaries, 79-80, 89, 93, 106-107, 235, 288

bowel movement, 85, 142, 147, 151, 154, 176
bowels, 85, 142, 147, 151, 154, 176, 269
Braille, 64
breasts, 38-39, 118, 149, 190, 260
breathing, 33-37, 117-119, 156, 158, 164, 167, 172, 175; and anxiety, 126; and arousal, 33; conscious, 34; difficulty, 6, 33, 129-130, 145; and orgasm, 137; Tantric, 34, 223-225, 227, 230-231, 233; and yoga, 226
Brent, Bill, 175
bulbar muscles, 44
butch, 333
butt plugs, 165, 198-200

C

caffeine, 142, 154
cancer, 260, 261
canes, 208, 246, 252, 255
caregivers, 32, 114, 151, 244, 274, 276-278, 280; *see also* personal care attendant
carpal tunnel syndrome, 63
catheters, 45, 81, 142, 148, 154, 182, 270, 277
centers for independent living, 98, 215
cerebral palsy (CP), 82, 141, 144-145, 172
cervical cancer, 261
cervix, 42-43
chanting, 226
chatrooms, 81, 82, 99, 100
chest pain, 129
China Brush, 209
chiropractors, 7
chlamydia, 258-259, 261, 283
chlorpromazine, 66
chlorthalidone, 66
chronic fatigue, 10-11, 29; *see also* fatigue
chronic pain, xi, 23, 49, 62, 80, 261; *see also* pain

cimetidine, 66
cisplain, 66
clamps, 207, 208, 253, 254
clitical.com, 123
clitoral stimulators, 217
clitoris, 31, 39-41, 43, 47, 52, 54, 58, 110, 135, 137, 148, 156-157, 159, 171, 173, 175, 203, 214, 217
clofibrate, 66
clonidine, 66
cocaine, 66
cock and ball torture, 254
cock rings, 202-203, 204, 268
coffee, 55, 142
cognitive disabilities, x, 9, 64, 278
collars, 207-208
colostomy, 82
Come as You Are, xi
coming out, 20-24
communication, 3, 51, 52, 63-64, 67, 69-109, 128, 135, 147, 151, 171, 187-188, 235-236, 241-242, 245, 246, 248, 252, 264, 279, 280, 285, 288; assistance with, 8; nonverbal, 64, 71, 86, 90-92, 125, 134, 140, 149, 156, 160, 176, 241; nonvisual, 125; with health care providers, 107-109; *see also* negotiation; augmentative and alternative communication; TTY
community, 18-19, 32, 225
computers, 98-99; hackers, 99; software, 98, 125
condoms, 31, 85, 143, 163, 176, 197, 204-205, 218-219, 220, 258-260, 261-266, 270-271, 273; assistance with, 105, 265; and catheters, 143; female, 219, 271; lubricated, 206; nonlatex, 219, 264, 270-271; polyurethane, 219, 270
consent, 72, 102, 138-139, 236, 238-240, 242, 254, 278, 289
contraceptives, *see* birth control
crabs, *see* pubic lice
creams, 208-209, 219-220
crops, 254

cross-dress, 139, 333
cunnilingus, 144, 152, 155-159, 177, 267
cybersex, 69, 81, 82, 98, 102, 114, 249
cystic fibrosis (CF), 145, 242-243

D

dancing, 10-11, 62, 73, 92
dating, 10, 18-19, 26, 62, 77, 81-83, 87-88, 90, 93-95, 97-100, 113, 125, 134, 145, 241, 249, 275, 279, 284
dating services, 97-100; online, 249
Delrin, 255
dental dams, 154, 176, 267
depression, 54, 64, 66-67, 129, 137, 147
Desikachar, Kausthub, 224-225
Desikachar, T. K. V., 224
desire, 13-15, 24, 53, 62, 63, 73, 74, 77, 79, 96, 101, 102, 106, 187, 212, 227, 244, 249, 255, 282, 288-289
developmental disabilities, x, 9, 278
devotees, 101
diabetes, 137, 146
diazepam, 66
digoxin, 66
dildos, 122, 162, 165, 170, 172-175, 176, 180, 187, 190, 196-198, 200-201, 215, 268; and allergies, 218-219; cleaning, 220; and gender play, 133; history, 271; realistic, 197; rubber, 197; silicone, 197-198, 219
disability community, xi, xii, 243
Disability Rag, The, ix
disability research, 57-58, 136
disability rights, 5
discharge, 258-259, 261
discipline, 239
disclosure, 81-84
dis-n-tangle, xi
diuretics, 66, 154
doctors, *see* physicians

Dodson, Betty, 58, 115
dominant, 239
doxipin, 66
drag queen, 333
Duncan, Gosnell, 271
Duncan, Kath, 101
Durex, 270
DVDs, 222

E

Easy for You to Say: Q&A's for Teens Living with Chronic Illness or Disability, xii
ejaculation, 53, 55-56, 59, 66, 142; in men, 45, 47, 55-56, 57, 116, 131, 137, 146, 149, 152, 163, 202, 209, 231-233, 266; in women, 41-42, 55, 143; retrograde, 56
email, 99, 100, 289
emotional health, 256
empowerment, xii, 20, 28, 57, 186-187, 235-236, 238, 242, 246
endocrine conditions, xii, 137
endometriosis, 10
endorphins 15, 247, 255
energy, 61, 62, 128-130, 151, 216, 225, 227, 228, 230
energy body, 228
environmental disabilities, x, 208
epilepsy, 146-147
erectile tissue, 41, 44, 46, 51, 54
erection, 39, 45, 53-54, 131, 148, 149, 173, 185, 200, 209; and cock rings, 202-203; difficulty with, 28, 85, 114, 130, 151; and medication, 66, 147; painful, 146; and penis pumps, 203-204; retrograde, 146
erotica, 211; *see also* books; pornography; videos
escort agencies, 103-104
Essential Tantra, The, 230
estrogen, 66
exhibitionists, 139
expectations, 14, 26, 51, 63-64, 73, 124, 126, 135, 148, 153-154, 230
EZ-On, 141, 264, 270

F

family, 5, 7, 12, 20, 22, 32, 70, 92-93, 115, 244, 248, 278-279
fantasy, 14, 51, 58, 63, 64, 65, 70, 75, 84, 109, 117-118, 120, 131-132, 133, 136, 169, 176, 186, 191, 200, 210, 229, 234-235, 245, 248-249, 251, 282
Fatale Media, 169
fatigue, 24-25, 62-63, 129, 146, 147, 260; and communication, 64, 76; and masturbation, 121; and negotiation, 252; and positions, 184; and safewords, 240; and sex toys, 213, 215-216; and sexual response, 144
feathers, 37-38, 119, 122, 134, 190, 207-208, 253-255
fellatio, 155, 159-163
femme, 333
fetishes, 101, 138-139, 249-250
films, 177
Finger Fitting Products, 214
finger fucking, 171
fisting, 171-172
flagellation, 208, 246-247
flashbacks, 241-242, 282, 285
flirting, 77, 86-90
floggers, 208, 216, 217, 220, 246-247, 253-254
foot fetish, 139
foreplay, 3, 63, 134, 154
foreskin, 45, 159-160, 265
frenulum, 45-46, 160
friction, 45, 119, 122, 148, 160
frotteurism, 139
FTM, 334
Fukuoku, 214

G

gays, 19-20, 22, 39, 92, 150, 210, 212, 291, 331, 333
gender, xi, 97, 106, 330-331; identity, 22, 30; play, 132-133, 139, 201, 245; roles, 147-148, 279
genital warts, 261

gloves, 170-171, 176, 218, 255, 267-268, 269-270
glycerin, 206, 209
gonorrhea, 259, 261, 283
Good Vibrations, 169
Grafenberg, Ernst, 42
Grant, Cameron, 213
group homes, 7
G-spot, 41-42, 48, 55, 58, 171, 175, 197

H

haloperidol, 66
handcuffs, 207, 243
harnesses, 133, 172, 174, 197, 200-201, 215
health insurance, 237, 264
hearing impairment, 9, 10
heart disease, 33, 125-126, 129-130
heart palpitations, 130
heart rate, 33, 51, 54, 57, 126, 137, 269, 282
hepatitis, 176, 258, 267, 283
herbalists, 7
heroin, 66
herpes, 259-260, 271, 283
heterosexuals, 22, 38-39, 169, 178, 212
hospices, 7
Hospital for Sick Children in Toronto, xii
Hotmail, 99
human immunodeficiency virus (HIV), 6, 165, 260-261, 267, 283; testing, 263-264
human papilloma virus (HPV), 261, 271, 283
hydralazine, 66
hypersensitivity, 139, 143-144, 217-218

I

identity, 18-24, 30, 71
immune system, 217, 218-220, 260-261
incontinence, 24, 55, 59, 139, 142-143, 147, 154,
infomercials, 72-73

insertion toys, 202, 217; *see also* sex
    toys
institutions, 7-8
intellectual disabilities, 9
International Professional Surrogates
    Association, 103
Internet, x, 32, 81, 98-100, 102, 111,
    188-189, 221, 222, 291
intersex, 22, 30, 332
intestinal parasites, 176, 261, 267
intimacy, 14, 23, 71, 85, 105, 150,
    168-169, 173, 230, 277; *see also*
    relationships
"It's Time to Politicize Our Sexual
    Oppression," ix

J
jackinworld.com, 123
joint pain, 177

K
Kaplan, Helen Singer, 53
Kegel excercises, 59-61
kidney disease, 129, 136-137
kissing, 3, 13, 67, 96, 145, 165-167,
    177, 178, 225, 241, 274, 284
Krishnamacharya, T., 224

L
labia, 39-41, 47
labia majora, 40
labia minora, 41
latex, 170, 255; and lubricants, 204;
    see also allergies
Latino, 20
leather community, *see* S/M
    community
lesbians, xi, 20, 22, 150, 177, 210,
    212, 279, 291, 331, 333
Lexan, 255
libido, 2, 61, 67
Liquid Silk, 205, 206
lotions, 208-209
lubricants, 122, 137, 146, 170-171,
    175, 176, 199, 202, 204-207, 265;
    and allergies, 206, 219, 269;

consistency, 205; ingredients,
    206-207; and latex, 204-205;
    oil-based, 204-205; research, 206;
    and rubber toys, 204-205; silicone-
    based, 204-205; and silicone toys,
    205; spermicidal, 271; taste, 154,
    205, 206; water-based, 137, 204-
    205; water-soluble, 205
lupus, 129

M
magazines, 73, 111, 205; erotic, 210;
    fashion, 48; fetish, 139
Maintain, 209
marijuana, 66
marital aids, 191
massage oil, 208-209, 219
massage therapists, 7
massage, 134, 231; erotic, 102;
    perineal, 45, 146, 232; prostate, 45
massagers, 192; *see also* vibrators
Masters, William and Johnson, Virginia,
    53
masturbation, 4, 31, 34, 48, 52, 62,
    63, 82, 110-123, 132, 137, 144,
    147, 184, 187, 188, 192, 232, 243,
    280, 282, 285; and self-esteem,
    15; and water, 62, 116, 119-120,
    122-123, 190; *see also* shower
    massager
mayerlabs.com, 264
media, 2, 67, 74, 177
medical establishment, 8, 68, 107,
    138, 229, 243, 264, 285
medical technicians, 276-277
medication, 39, 47, 129, 146, 147,
    216; and communication, 64, 108;
    and decreased lubrication, 137,
    204; and difficulty reaching orgasm,
    59, 66; and erection, 54, 173, 204;
    and masturbation, 120; and
    negotiation, 250; and reduced
    libido, 65-67, 144; *see also*
    antidepressants
mental health, 256
methadone, 66

methyl paraben, 206
methyldopa, 66
milk-producing tissue, 39
mobility concerns, 29, 63, 139-140,
    144, 216, 286; and positions, 184;
    and sex toys, 213, 214-215; and
    S/M, 246; *see also* accessibility
mobility disability, xi, 29, 101
monogamy, 333
Montegue, Ashley, 133
Morgan, Robert, 169
Morin, Jack, 174
MTF, 334
multiple-chemical sensitivities, 218-220
multiple sclerosis (MS), 9, 10, 147-148
muscular dystrophy (MD), 172
myths, 2-12, 72-73

N

naproxen, 66
National Spinal Cord Injury
    Foundation, 271
naturopaths, 7
negative beliefs, 12, 14, 16, 29, 52,
    55, 73, 91, 255
negotiation, with attendants, 104-107;
    with partners, 83, 200; in S/M, 236,
    250-252
neurological conditions, 58, 141
newsgroups, 99-100
newspaper, 72-73, 103
Night Rider, 201
nipple clamps, 208, 254
nipples, 38-39, 54, 116, 118, 148;
    stimulation, 28, 38-39, 120, 122,
    136, 145, 160, 165, 203, 208, 209,
    254
nitrile, 268
nitrous oxide, 66
nondisabled people, x-xi, 5, 9, 10, 22,
    31, 56-58, 63, 73-83, 85, 94, 114,
    136, 201, 211, 228, 246, 281, 285
nonlatex supplies, 219, 264, 267-268,
    270-271
nonlatex toys, 272
nonmonogamy, 237

nonoxynol-9, 206, 260
nurses, 31, 277
nursing homes, 7, 114
NutraSweet, 206

O

O'Brien, Mark, 103
occipital nerve, 116
occupational therapist, 215
online discussion groups, 250; *see also*
    Internet
oral sex, 3, 84, 102, 145, 150-167,
    174, 184, 260, 264, 267, 274, 284;
    see also cunnilingus; fellatio; kissing
orgasm, 4, 33, 41, 43, 52-59, 66, 95,
    111, 113, 114, 119, 120, 121, 129,
    134-138, 142, 143, 146, 147, 148,
    155, 158, 159, 169, 189-190, 227-
    229, 231-233, 275, 282-283,
    285-286; and anal penetration,
    175; and cervical stimulation, 58,
    121; clitoral, 58; dry, 56; extended,
    59; G-spot, 42, 58; multiple, 2, 53,
    57-58; nonejaculatory, 57, 232-
    233; phantom, 136; relaxation, 58;
    simultaneous, 3; tension, 58;
    vaginal, 58; whole body, 59, 126
ostomies, 95, 139, 143

P

paddles, 208, 217, 235, 254
pain, 7, 10, 15, 17, 23, 24-25, 32, 37,
    45, 47, 67, 76, 123, 127, 129, 133,
    137, 157, 162, 175, 215, 257, 259,
    260, 261, 262, 270, 282, 286-287;
    and arousal, 52, 54; and breathing,
    34; and communication, 76, 84,
    91-92, 96; and erection, 146; and
    masturbation, 63, 115-116, 120,
    121; menstrual, 137; and orgasm,
    56, 66, 175; and penetration, 121,
    142, 170, 204; and pleasure, 112,
    208, 235, 242-244, 247, 254; and
    positions, 61-62, 159, 177-178,
    180; research, 62; and self-care,
    24-25; and self-esteem, 17; and sex

toys, 215-216; and sexual response, 49, 51, 52, 61-62, 145; and yoga, 225-226; *see also* chronic pain
palpitations, 130
pansexual, 333
Pap smear, 31, 261
paraplegic, 116, 119
partners, 124-149; and abuse, 280; choosing, 93, 287; and coercion, 256, 272-273; cyber, 98-100; disabled, 93-94; finding, 20-21, 30, 86-90, 92-104, 248-250; and masturbation 121-122; nondisabled, xi; and oral sex, 150-151, 153, 154, 158-159, 163; people with disabilities as, 1, 4-5, 14-15, 29; and porn, 211-212; and self-esteem, 30; and STIs, 263; *see also* communication
passing, 22
Patanjali, 223-224
PC muscle, *see* pubococcygeal muscle
PCA, *see* personal care attendant
PCP, 66
pelvic inflammatory disease (PID), 261-262, 263
penetration, 134-135, 137, 169-183; anal, 164, 174-176; and arthritis, 144; and catheters, 143; and cerebral palsy, 142; and cervical stimulation, 148; with dildos, 172-174; with fingers, 170-171; fisting, 171; and masturbation, 122; and oral sex, 156; and orgasm, 58; and ostomies, 143; painful, 170; with penises, 148, 173-174; with sex toys, 165; and spasticity, 140-141; and spinal cord injury, 148; vaginal, 82, 135, 141, 165, 169-174; *see also* positions
penis, 28, 39, 44-46, 47, 54, 59, 114, 135, 137, 143, 152, 155, 159-163, 168-169, 173-174, 201-204, 209, 214, 217, 232, 265-266, 330-332; circumcised, 45, 159-160; glans, 45-46; shaft, 45; uncircumcised, 159-160, 265

penis pumps, 173, 203-204
performance anxiety, 113, 225
perineum, 45
personal ads, 82, 97-100, 103, 249; online, 100, 249
personal care attendant (PCA), 8, 85, 104-107, 108-109, 116, 132-133, 257; and abuse, 275, 276-277; and masturbation, 116, 120-121; and partners, 77, 94-95, 104, 106; and privacy, 114; and safer sex, 265, 271; and STIs, 261; *see also* caregiver
pharmacology, 66-67
phone sex, 102
physical health, 256
physical therapists, 129, 192
physicians, 7, 17, 31, 39, 49, 56, 59, 65, 67-68, 73, 107-109, 115, 129, 137, 154, 169, 173-174, 188, 204, 244, 257, 263, 277
piercing, 238, 255
Planned Parenthood of Toronto, xi
pleasure, xii, 4, 23, 29, 38, 48-49, 51-52, 55-58, 62, 110-111, 112-113, 115, 116, 124, 126, 186-187, 209, 229, 235, 246, 282-283, 285
polyamory, 333
pony play, 139
pornography, 3, 111, 163, 210, 211-213; depictions of people with disabilities, 210-211; *see also* books; erotica; videos
positions, 85, 96, 129, 130, 140-141, 142, 143, 144, 145, 148, 151, 176-184, 205, 215; and analingus, 164; and blood pressure, 269; and cunnilingus, 158; doggie, 178; and fellatio, 160-161; and furniture, 183; and kissing, 165-166; missionary, 178; partner on top, 179-180; and pillows, 214; and sex toys, 216; side-by-side, 182-183; sixty-nine, 163-164; and S/M, 252-253; and wheelchairs, 180-181

post-traumatic stress disorder (PTSD), 49, 241-242
prazosin, 66
pregnancy, xi, 39, 127, 256, 263, 283; tubal, 259, 261
privacy, 7-8, 98, 287; and communication, 74-75, 90, 105, 106; and fantasy, 249; and masturbation, 113, 114-115, 117, 121; and sex toys, 217-218; and sexual health, 257, 263-264; and sexual response, 64- 65
Probe, 206
progesterone, 66
propranalol, 66
propyl paraben, 206
prostate, 46-47
prosthesis, penile, 152
prostitution, see sex work
psychiatric disabilities, x, 14, 236
psychological play, 235, 247-248, 253, 255
pubic lice, 262
pubococcygeal muscle (PC), 59, 61, 66, 173, 232

Q
quadriplegics, 16, 57, 63, 82, 111
Queen, Carol, 47, 169
queer, xi, 212, 291, 333

R
racism, 211
Ramses, 270
rashes, 209, 219, 260, 262, 270
Reality, 271
rectal cancer, 261
rectum, 47
reflexology, 134
refractory period, 57
rehab hospitals, 7
relationships, 4-5, 11, 15, 24, 71, 72, 75-84, 93-96, 131, 134, 212, 243, 264, 273, 275, 278-280, 284, 287-288; see also intimacy
respiratory system, 35

restraints, 207, 235, 245-246, 254
retrograde ejaculation, see ejaculation
rimming, see analingus
risk, 9, 30, 32, 93, 147, 164, 170, 197, 216, 220, 236, 256-257, 260-261, 263-265, 270, 276-278, 279
Royalle, Candida, 213

S
sadomasochism, 235
safer sex, 85, 102, 164, 170, 176, 198, 219, 220-221, 256-275
safety, 102, 133, 188, 197, 238, 241, 256, 273, 286-287
safewords, 91-92, 240-241, 250-251
scar tissue, 28-29
Scorpio Products, 271
scrotum, 44-46, 162, 174, 202, 214
selective serotonin reuptake inhibitor (SSRI), 66-67
self-care, 24-25
self-esteem, 15-26
self-image, 15, 20, 21
self-monitoring, 7, 198, 220-221, 247, 251, 257-258
self-pleasuring, see masturbation
sensation, 28, 32, 37-39, 42, 126, 139-140, 147, 148, 149, 152, 166, 175, 176, 230-231, 232-233, 234, 242, 244, 246, 247, 254, 255, 257, 267-268, 287; genital, 45, 47, 143, 144, 160, 164, 169; and orgasm, 56, 57, 59, 136, 148; and sexual response, 51-53, 54; and medication, 65-67; and masturbation, 116, 117, 122; and sex toys, 188, 198-199, 202-203, 207-208, 209, 216-217, 218, 220; and touch, 134; see also hypersensitivity
sensory control, 244
sensory deprivation, 207
sensory disabilities, x
sex education, 29, 31, 64, 74, 103, 169, 175, 206, 210,
sex educators, xi-xii, 9, 33, 47, 48, 55, 111, 112, 154, 167, 169, 242, 267

Sex for One, 115
sex research, x, 4, 48-49, 53, 54, 55, 56, 299
sex therapist, 170
sex toy stores, 74, 112, 189, 210, 213, 218, 221-222
sex toys, 62, 74, 149, 156-157, 185-222; accessibility, 112, 114, 201; adapting, xi, 213; and allergies, 218-219, 269-272; anal, 165, 169, 176, 198-200; bondage, 207; buying, 221-222; cleaning, 195, 217-219; and fantasy, 118-119; and fatigue, 215-216; G-spot, 42; Kegel, 61; and mobility, 214-215; and motor control, 214-215; for men, 45, 47, 174, 201-204; and oral sex, 156, 165; and orgasm, 121, 189-190; for penetration, 169-170, 177; and positions, 140, 184; and safer sex, 220-221; and safety, 268-269; sensation, 207-208; S/M, 207-208, 234, 244, 254-255; *see also* specific toys
sex work, 48, 100-104
SexAbility, xi
sexism, 211
sexual abuse, 8-9, 115, 187, 274-289; *see also* sexual assault
sexual aids, 191
sexual arousal, 22, 33, 42-43, 48-54, 57, 58, 63, 111-112, 141, 146, 147, 149, 209, 210, 232, 282; and ejaculation, 232; and erection, 203; and fantasy, 131, 152; and fetishes, 139; and lubrication, 137, 170
sexual assault, 8-9, 105, 137, 274-289; research, 276; *see also* sexual abuse
sexual desire, 77
sexual identity, 19, 212
sexual independence, xii
sexual need, 77
sexual response, 9, 28, 30, 48-68, 74, 103, 113, 138, 189, 190, 217, 229, 232, 283, 289

sexual response cycle, 49, 53; desire, 53; excitement, 53, 228; plateau, 53; orgasm, 53, 228; resolution, 53
sexual surrogates, 103
sexual vocabulary, 74
sexualhealth.com, 229
sexually transmitted disease (STD), 256, 257, 258, 263
sexually transmitted infection (STI), 170, 220, 258-263, 266-267, 270, 283
Sheiks, 270
Shiatsu, 134
shower massager, 119-120, 190
silicone, 195-198, 219, 220, 271, 272; and lubricants, 204-205
slapping, 174, 245, 246
sling, 184
Slippery Stuff, 206
S/M, 91-92, 102, 139, 207-208, 210, 234-255; bottom, 239; community, 235-238, 243, 249-250; top, 239
soft drinks, 142
Spanish Fly, 209
spanking, 6, 242, 245, 246, 251, 252, 254-255
spasms, 34, 49-50, 52, 139, 140-142, 149, 170, 207, 214, 232, 242
spasticity, 140-141, 144, 147, 151, 178, 269
speech therapists, 71
speed, 66
spinal cord, 54
spinal cord injury (SCI), 9, 56-58, 121, 136, 141, 147-149, 229, 269, 271
spironolactone, 66
spontaneity, 3, 16, 72, 125, 126, 127-128, 131, 235-236
spronolactone, 66
Sta-hard, 209
stereotypes, 20, 70, 111,148, 236, 238
sterility, 258, 261
Stormy Leather, 201
strap-ons, 133, 172, 174, 177
stress, 127, 130, 137, 177, 232, 260, 286; and masturbation, 114, 118, 200
strip clubs, 102

stroke, 9, 125, 149
Stubbs, Kenneth Ray, 230
Stud 100, 209
stuffing, 173-174
submissive, 239
support, 32
sweat glands, 153
syphilis, 262

T

taboo, 4, 174, 176, 248
talk radio, 48, 72-73
Tantra, 34, 223-233, 239
Taormino, Tristan, 175
tea, 55, 142
temperature play, 122, 209, 255, 231
temporarily able-bodied (TAB), 78
Tepper, Mitch, 56-57, 229
testicles, 45-46, 57, 61, 160, 162, 259, 330
Thai beads, 199
therapists, 7, 103, 187, 282
Thomas, Paul, 213
thoracic level, 6
tickling, 122, 148-149, 190, 208, 254, 331
timing, 63, 81, 84, 85, 127, 143, 216
timolol, 66
touch, 128, 132, 133-134, 138, 139, 140, 143, 160, 167, 173, 204, 208, 217, 282, 284-285, 287; and abuse, 274-275; and caregivers, 151, 277; and communication, 77, 89, 125; and masturbation, 111, 115, 116, 120; and positions, 176, 180, 182; and sexual response, 28, 31, 37-39, 41-42, 45, 48, 50-51; and S/M, 235, 239, 244-245, 252; and timing, 127
transgender, xi, 22, 291, 333
transitioning, 334
transsexual, xi, 22, 30, 291, 333-334
transvestite, 139, 333
trauma 32, 113, 115, 132, 281-283, 286; see also post-traumatic stress disorder

trichomonas, 262-263
Trojan Supra, 270-271
trust, xi, 93, 95-96, 104, 114, 168-169, 171, 187, 204, 225, 237-238, 245, 263-264, 275, 279, 282-284
TTD, 222
TTY, 32, 222, 289
TV, 12, 72-74, 111, 177

U

Ultimate Guide to Anal Sex for Men, The, 175
Ultimate Guide to Anal Sex for Women, The, 174-175
urethra, 39-41, 44-46, 146, 157, 330
urethral sponge, *see* G-spot
urination, 28, 41, 45, 55, 59, 143, 144, 258-259, 260, 263, 266
urologists, 174
uterus, 42-43

V

vagina, 39-43, 54, 57, 59-61, 119, 130, 135, 136-137, 143, 145; lubrication, 137, 145, 148, 152, 169-170, 171, 209, 220, 283; *see also* penetration
vaginismus, 170
Vedas, 223
ventilator, 34
vestibular glands, 41
vibrators, 119, 122, 147, 187, 192-196, 201, 202, 217, 221, 269; "addiction" to, 188; and allergies, 218; assistance with, 105, 116; battery-powered, 194-196, 218; butterfly, 144; cleaning, 105; coil, 194, 218; egg, 119; electric, 192-194, 218; and fatigue, 216; insertable, 42; and motor control, 148, 214; and oral sex, 155, 165; and orgasm, 146, 189-190; and plastic, 195; and positions, 177; and privacy, 217-218; rubber, 195; silicone, 195, 271; wand, 194; waterproof, 214, 218

videos, porn, 116, 211-213, 221, 222; fetish, 139
Viniyoga, 224-225
viruses, 258, 259-261, 264, 283
visual impairment, 125
voyeurs, 139
vulva, 39-40

W

wax, 253, 255
Waxman, Barbara Faye, ix
wheelchairs, 6, 8, 18, 24, 28, 92, 101, 118, 128, 131, 180-181, 201, 211, 250-251; and accessibility, 237; and Night Rider harness, 201; and porn, 211; and positions, 148, 161, 166, 181; and public sex, 130

Whipple, Beverley, 48, 136, 229
whips, 208, 216, 217, 220, 235, 243, 245, 246-247, 254
World Wide Web, 98; *see also* Internet

Y

Yahoo, 99
yeast infections, 146, 206, 220, 258
yoga, 223-226
Yoga Sutras, 223-224

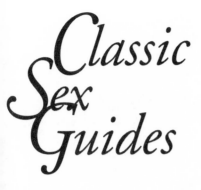

Classic Sex Guides

THE GOOD VIBRATIONS GUIDE TO SEX

THE MOST COMPLETE SEX MANUAL EVER WRITTEN

Third Edition

Cathy Winks and Anne Semans
Illustrated by Phoebe Gloeckner

"Useful for absolutely everyone. Old, young, fit, disabled, gay, straight or working out the details, this book tells you, shows you and reassures you."—*O, The Oprah Magazine*

$25.95   ISBN 1-57344-158-9

THE WHOLE LESBIAN SEX BOOK

A PASSIONATE GUIDE FOR ALL OF US

Felice Newman

"The most complete, all-questions-answered, savvy guide to lesbian, butch, bisexual, femme, androgynous and trans-gendered sex! Keep it next to your bed!"—*Good Vibrations*

"Superb. Why can't more heterosexual sex manuals be this good?"—*Library Journal*

$24.95   ISBN 1-57344-088-4

SENSUOUS MAGIC

A GUIDE FOR ADVENTUROUS COUPLES

Second Edition

Patrick Califia

This much-loved beginner's guide to S/M for couples is for all readers who harbor fantasies of erotic dominance and submission. Completely revised and updated, featuring all-new erotic stories by Califia.

$14.95   ISBN 1-57344-130-9

THE SURVIVOR'S GUIDE TO SEX

HOW CREATE YOUR OWN EMPOWERED SEXUALITY AFTER CHILDHOOD SEXUAL ABUSE

Staci Haines

The first encouraging, sex-positive guide for all women survivors of sexual assault.

"What a terrific book! Every survivor needs this encouraging, down-to-earth guide— and the joy of freely-chosen, healthy sexual pleasure."—*Ellen Bass*

$24.95   ISBN 1-57344-079-5

Bestselling sex guides from Cleis Press are available from your favorite bookseller.
Cleis Press • (800) 780-2279 • www.cleispress.com

The "Best" Erotica Series...

BEST WOMEN'S EROTICA SERIES

Edited by Marcy Sheiner

"Gets racier every year."—*San Francisco Bay Guardian*

Sexy, smart and literate—these erotic stories are for readers who want to know the truth about women's sexuality in all its variety and emotional depth, with all of its surprises and twists and turns.

BEST WOMEN'S EROTICA 2004
ISBN 1-57344-181-3 $14.95

BEST WOMEN'S EROTICA 2003
ISBN 1-57344-160-0 $14.95

BEST WOMEN'S EROTICA 2002
ISBN 1-57344-141-4 $14.95

BEST WOMEN'S EROTICA 2001
ISBN 1-57344-117-1 $14.95

BEST WOMEN'S EROTICA
ISBN 1-57344-099-X $14.95

BEST BLACK WOMEN'S EROTICA SERIES

Real black women's sexuality in all of its fullness and variety.

"Exciting, humorous, and quite a resource of sensual navigation."—*Terry McMillan*

BEST BLACK WOMEN'S EROTICA
Edited by Blanche Richardson
ISBN 1-57344-106-6 $14.95

BEST BLACK WOMEN'S EROTICA 2
Edited by Samiya Bashir
ISBN 1-57344-163-5 $14.95

BEST BONDAGE EROTICA

Edited by Alison Tyler
ISBN 1-57344-173-2 $14.95

BEST BISEXUAL WOMEN'S EROTICA

Edited by Cara Bruce
ISBN 1-57344-134-1 $14.95

BEST FETISH EROTICA

Edited by Cara Bruce
ISBN 1-57344-146-5 $14.95

Bestselling erotica from Cleis Press is available from your favorite bookseller.
Cleis Press • (800) 780-2279 • www.cleispress.com